Nutrition and Global Health

Nutrition and Global Health

Shawn W. McLaren
Lecturer
London Metropolitan University
England, United Kingdom

WILEY Blackwell

This edition first published 2023
© 2023 John Wiley & Sons Ltd

The right of Shawn W. McLaren to be identified as the author of the editorial material in this work has been asserted in accordance with law.

Registered Office
John Wiley & Sons, Inc., 111 River Street, Hoboken, NJ 07030, USA
John Wiley & Sons Ltd, The Atrium, Southern Gate, Chichester, West Sussex, PO19 8SQ, UK

Editorial Office
9600 Garsington Road, Oxford, OX4 2DQ, UK

For details of our global editorial offices, customer services and more information about Wiley products visit us at www.wiley.com.

Wiley also publishes its books in a variety of electronic formats and by print-on-demand. Some content that appears in standard print versions of this book may not be available in other formats.

Library of Congress Cataloging-in-Publication data applied for
Paperback ISBN: 9781119779827

Cover Design: Wiley
Cover Image: © Riccardo Niels Mayer/Adobe Stock Photos

Set in 11.5/13.5pt STIXTwoText by Straive, Pondicherry, India
Printed and bound by CPI Group (UK) Ltd, Croydon, CR0 4YY

C9781119779827_260922

Contents

Preface

*N*utrition and Global Health began some years ago as a series of short literature reviews. Many of my lectures begin as short literature reviews, written in full, to help to organise my thoughts and identify the key sources and ideas for a given topic. Over time, these notes became too large and detailed to fully cover in a lecture, so when Wiley contacted me, I immediately started work on converting those lecture notes into this textbook. Global health is a vast topic – it is quite literally global. It involves all kinds of clinicians, policymakers, planners, patients and populations. When I began teaching a university module on nutrition in the global health context, I quickly recognised that, while there are excellent textbooks already available, I could not find one that captured nutrition and global health in the way that I would like to understand and teach it. Nutrition is often integrated into other disciplines; it is an important aspect of many interventions, and the success of interventions can be supported by good nutrition practices. Nutrition is an applied science, but it has its basis in biochemistry, human physiology, behavioural science and even political studies. These divisions are present in many of the textbooks which are available to students and practitioners. It is easy to find the recommended action for a given challenge in a global health context, but the rationale for the action is often less obvious and needs to be sought elsewhere. Sometimes an action is recommended but some additional thought and guidance are needed to work out how the action can be implemented. There are many useful resources available to the student or practitioner in global health and nutrition, but these are often long and complex policy documents, and a fuller understanding of these documents relies on a solid foundation in more basic sciences. Therefore, the purpose of this book is to provide students and practitioners with a roadmap for interpreting the global health landscape, and to create links between nutritional physiology, policy and action. I have drawn extensively on the available literature as well of my own experience of working in the field. I qualified as a dietitian and worked in clinical and public health settings before moving into academia. Among the questions I had in the early stages of my career were "how do I design an effective intervention?" and "how can I decide whether or not my intervention has done what I intended it to do?". I have included opportunities for developing the reader's analytic skills throughout this book, based on widely used practices in global health. I hope this book helps readers become more effective practitioners in global health and supports their studies in this exciting and critically important field.

Shawn W. McLaren

1

Introduction

The medical model of health as the 'absence of disease' can be traced back as far as the ancient Greeks. The definition of health adopted by the World Health Organisation in 1948 (WHO 1948) refers to health as a state of complete physical, mental and social well-being, and not merely the absence of disease or infirmity. The emphasis therefore changed to health as well-being. However, Huber et al. (2011) have challenged the WHO definition of health, considering it no longer fit for purpose. The Ottawa Charter for Health Promotion (WHO 1987) defines health as a resource. The definition is given as 'health is a resource for everyday life, not the object of living. It is a positive concept emphasising social and personal resources as well as physical capabilities'. Building on this definition, Huber et al. (2011) suggest that the emphasis in defining health should be placed on the ability to adapt and self-manage in the face of social, physical and emotional challenges. The global population is becoming increasingly aware of the importance of health as a resource. Economists model future projections of growth and stability on the health and well-being of the population. Health and nutritional status affect mental development, years of schooling a child receives, and can even predict changes in IQ, which can have important ramifications for economic activity and potential lifetime earnings. Being unable to work due to chronic or short-term illness costs individuals opportunities and earnings. Most importantly, health can impact quality of life.

Nutrition is 'The process of providing or obtaining food necessary for health and growth' (Oxford English Dictionary). Nutrition science is the investigation of the metabolic and physiological responses of the body to diet. Nutrition is an area of scientific enquiry that continues to grow. Research traditionally looked at sustaining life and preventing disease. The focus has shifted toward optimising health and life. Nutrition science draws on identifying nutrients and other compounds in food and drink.

Nutrition and Global Health, First Edition. Shawn W. McLaren.
© 2023 John Wiley & Sons Ltd. Published 2023 by John Wiley & Sons Ltd.

Hippocrates (fifth century BCE), the ancient Greek physician, dedicated his treatise 'On diet' to the presentation of his nutritional concepts and the role of diet in the treatment of diseases. 'Flesh is added to his flesh and bones to his bones, and in the same way the appropriate thing is added to each of his other parts' (Phaedo 96C ± D and The Statesman 288E ± 289A). In The Republic, he added that 'the first and chief of our needs is the provision of food for existence and life'. Plato (fifth century BCE) was also interested in diet, and his writings on diet and nutrition recommended moderating the amount of meat and wine that people consumed, while recommending cereals, legumes, fish, fruits, milk and honey – not unlike an ancient form of what became known in the twentieth century as the Mediterranean diet (Skiadas and Lascaratos 2001).

There was a fundamental shift in the thought behind the causes of disease and death in the nineteenth century. Prior to the emergence of germ theory, public health science was dominated by miasmatic theory. Miasma theory held that illness was caused by 'miasma', the foul smell arising from rotting organic matter. During the Black Death in the sixteenth century, plague doctors would wear masks stuffed with sweet herbs in order to protect themselves from the disease-carrying smells. It also meant that public health efforts were focused on adequate waste disposal and hygiene. The principles of hygiene and cleanliness were adopted successfully by Florence Nightingale during the Crimean war, which aided in reducing the mortality rate in field hospitals by two-thirds. Nightingale (1859) was also an early proponent of diet as an essential component of clinical treatment, stating 'thousands of patients are annually starved in the midst of plenty from want of attention to the ways which make it possible for them to take food. I say to the nurse, have a rule of thought about your patient's diet'. Around the same time, the theory that specific living organisms were responsible for spreading disease was growing. During the cholera outbreak in London 1850s, John Snow demonstrated that cholera was transmitted through water that had been contaminated by the faeces of cholera patients and had the water pump in Soho closed.

Early investigations into nutrition were also made during the Victorian period. Quatelet, a French mathematician, first described an index that could be used to assess body weight in relation to height. Quatelet's index was largely forgotten until the 1970s, when it resurfaced and was renamed the body mass index (BMI).

Louis Pasteur proved the germ theory – that pathogenic microorganisms were responsible for causing illness – in the nineteenth century. Once this theory was adopted by medicine in the 1880s, it became the predominant line of thought amongst clinicians in treating diseases. However, it was soon discovered that not all ailments could be explained or linked to specific pathogens. Traditional approaches to health, which often focused on balance between the needs of people and the environment, were supressed during the colonial period, and replaced with biomedical approaches to public health (Loewenson et al. 2021).

Evidence for micronutrient deficiency originated in the early 1800s, when a French scientist named Francious Magendie recognised that malnourished dogs developed corneal ulcerations. These were symptoms of vitamin A deficiency; however, the compound responsible for preventing the deficiency state was not discovered until the early decades of the twentieth century. The requirement for thiamine was recognised in the late 1800s when fowl fed on a diet of cooked, polished rice developed neurological problems that presented in a similar way to beriberi. This discovery took place in Indonesia, by army physician Christiaan Eijkman, who was engaged in studying malaria at the time. When the mess officer realised that Eijkman was feeding his fowls the polished rice, he refused to supply more, stating that he would not have chickens eating rice from the mess as they were not commissioned officers. This meant that Eijkman had to return to feeding the chickens unpolished rice, and he noticed that the neurological symptoms resolved themselves. The observation led Eijkman to infer that something essential was contained in the husks of rice, which was required for normal function of the nervous system. After some time investigating, thiamine was isolated, a discovery that earned him the Nobel prize in 1901.

The early decades of the twentieth century saw the isolation of the rest of the vitamins, often by painstaking trial and error experiments. Different dietary components were investigated to find compounds that were essential to health. The Burrs fed rats on a highly controlled fat-free diet and observed their physiological response. The rats developed dry, scaly skin and poor growth compared with rats who were given the same diet with additional cod-liver oil (Burr and Burr 1929). Specific fats were later reintroduced, and the rat's recovery was reported; however, recovery was dependent on the combination of fats given, implying that some specific fatty acids had a role to play in skin health and growth. These were later isolated and identified as omega-3 and omega-6 fatty acids. All the remaining major vitamins were isolated during the 1920s to 1940s, e.g. vitamin A, vitamins B1 to B12, vitamins C, D, E and K. During this time, spurred by the Great Depression and World War II, guidelines were developed for total calorie intake and selected nutrients. Governments were particularly interested in nutritional status, food intakes and health during this period as rationing took hold during the second world war. Careful analysis was required in order to ensure that the population would receive adequate nutrition, while limiting and preventing waste as far as possible.

Although it has been speculated that the symptoms of kwashiorkor were described in medicine as early as Hippocrates (Adams 1849), malnutrition only became a focus of medical research during the early twentieth century (Trowell and Davies 1952). It had been noted that kwashiorkor was most prevalent amongst infants during the weaning phase and could be linked to the poor quality of complementary foods (Trowell and Davies 1952). The term kwashiorkor comes from a Ghanaian Kwa word linking the birth order of a child to illness. A second child is born, and the first-born is weaned and changed to a starchy, nutrient-poor cereal, thus developing the features of malnutrition. The term kwashiorkor was first used to describe this phenomenon in 1933 by Cicely D. Williams, and it was thought that the condition was the result of inadequate protein but approximately adequate energy intake. Williams described this condition in children eating diets based on maize that were high in carbohydrate but low in protein. The term 'protein energy malnutrition' was introduced by Jellie in 1959 but has since been replaced by the term acute malnutrition.

Initially, the index weight-for-age (WFA) was introduced to quantify growth retardation and had important consequences for health and policy planning (Gopolan and Rao 1984). Subsequently, Waterlow introduced the terms 'wasting' and 'stunting' to assist in differentiating types of growth retardation (Gopolan and Rao 1984). These terms have been adopted by the World Health Organisation.

Understanding of the physiology of acute malnutrition was improved substantially during the second world war. While working on the effects of high altitudes on human physiology after the outbreak of WWII, scientist Ancel Keys was pulled from his work by the Quartermaster Corps of the US Defence Department to advise on food for paratroopers. 'I knew nothing about diets then, and my interest in food was confined to good cooking and good eating' (Keys 1990). The only nutritional criterion for the paratrooper ration was total calories, and the combination of a hard piece of sausage, dry biscuits, a block of chocolate and a stick of chewing gum became known as the 'K-ration' and was the general combat ration for all US troops.

Towards the end of the war, it became apparent that nutritional rehabilitation would be necessary for people living in famine-hit regions and the survivors of concentration camps. The Minnesota experiment was not the first prospective trial on human starvation, but it remains the most famous. The experiment was designed and implemented by Keys and his colleagues in 1944, enlisting 36 conscientious objectors who followed a strictly controlled calorie reduction diet paired with a physical exercise regimen. Participants' food intake, exercise, biomarkers, anthropometric measurements and psychological states were monitored throughout the experiment. An important aspect of the Minnesota experiment is that participants were monitored through their rehabilitation phase. The results of this never-to-be-repeated study greatly increased our understanding of the effects of acute malnutrition in human beings. Findings regarding malnutrition and rehabilitation were used to inform aid workers' practice in Europe. Some of the advice given in the guidebook produced included to 'show no partiality, and refrain from arguments; the starving are ready to argue on little provocation, but they usually regret it immediately' and 'informing the group what is being done, and why, is just as important as getting things done – billboards are the easiest way'. When it came to eating arrangements, aid workers were advised that 'starvation increases the need for privacy and quiet – noise of all kinds seems to be very bothersome and especially so during mealtimes' and that 'energy is a commodity to be hoarded – living and eating quarters should be arranged conveniently'. The guidebook went on to suggest that since the starving are emotionally affected by the weather, cheerful activities could be saved for poor weather.

During the 1950s and 1960s, nutrition policy and agricultural technology focused on increasing staple calories and selected micronutrients. The 'green industrial revolution' took place during the second half of the twentieth century, which ushered in an era of industrial scale farming (Raven and Wagner 2021). A debate began over the role of fat and sugar in causing disease – the health risks of eating fats won scientific and policy support, but the debate continues today. Scientists disagreed on whether protein or total calories were most relevant in infant and young child feeding in developing nations. Industry created and promoted protein-enriched formulas in these regions.

It was also during the latter half of the twentieth century that an interest in identifying associations between mortality risk and overnutrition became an area of focus (Mozaffarian et al. 2018). Actuaries were interested in seeing whether it was a 'safe bet' to insure people with overweight and obesity. Keys had previously identified the problem inherent in nutritional and health surveys from the early twentieth century – that many of these surveys collected data on weight only, making them difficult to interpret. Many anthropometric measures of nutritional status were suggested, including identifying a reference weight and calculating overweight as a percentage of the reference weight. During the 1970s, Keys coined the term 'body mass index', which described the earlier Quatelet's index. This marked a resurgence of the use of BMI, which continues to be used to monitor the health and nutritional status of populations and individuals today.

Dietary guidelines shifted emphasis on high-income nations from preventing deficiencies to preventing chronic disease during the 1980s. The world began to work in partnership to eliminate hunger and nutritional deficiencies in lower income countries, implementing widespread aid, micronutrient supplementation and fortification strategies. By 2000, it was becoming more apparent that dietary patterns played a larger role in chronic diseases than single nutrients did. A rapid rise in chronic diseases all over the world led to the recognition of the 'double burden of disease', simultaneous nutrient deficiency along with increased rates of diabetes, cardiovascular disease, obesity, and cancer. There is growing concern for environmental and health effects of modern crop farming, livestock practices, additives and how we will feed a growing population with finite resources.

There was an interesting change of paradigm that took place towards the end of the twentieth century. Shifts in political power and superpowers resulted in a change in emphasis from 'international health' towards 'global health'. International health can be conceived as the relationships between individual nations, primarily focused on their own public health, such as controlling infectious diseases crossing borders. Global health emerged from international health during an era of increasing velocity of globalisation, when it was recognised that the health concerns of the entire global population are interconnected and that the effects of events such as climate change and global pandemics are not limited to individual nations (Brown et al. 2006). There has also been growing recognition that traditional socio-cultural approaches are required on the world stage in order to address current challenges in global health (Loewenson et al. 2021).

The Millennium Development Goals (MDGs) were developed by the United Nations (UN) in 2000 with the intention of providing a basis for local government policies. The MDGs helped to coordinate international aid to focus on eight areas for development in an overarching global development framework. The eight MDGs were to eradicate extreme poverty and hunger, achieve universal primary education, promote gender equality and empower women, reduce child mortality, improve maternal health, combat HIV/AIDS, malaria, and other diseases, ensure environmental sustainability and develop a global partnership for development. MDG 1, to eradicate extreme poverty and hunger, included objective 1.C – to halve the number of people suffering from hunger between 1990 and 2015. Hunger was measured using parameters including child stunting, access to adequate food around the year, sustainable food systems, smallholder productivity and a reduction in food waste. In 1990–1992, there were 991 million undernourished people worldwide, representing 23.3% of the global population. The figure had reduced to 902 million people or 18.3% of the population in 1999–2001. In 2015, 10.6% of the global population was undernourished, corresponding to 785.4 million people. The UN considered this target as having been met as the proportion of people who were undernourished had been halved. However, in absolute terms, the number of people suffering from hunger had only reduced by 205 million or 20.7% as the world population continued to increase during the MDG period. In 2018, 10.8% or 821 million people were undernourished.

The Sustainable Development Goals (SDGs) replaced the MDGs in 2015. Agencies involved in the development and implementation of the SDGs include the World Food Programme, World Health Organisation, World Bank, Food and Agriculture Organisation of the UN (FAO) and International Fund for Agricultural Development. Nutrition plays a role in achieving the aims of promoting economic development, improvements in literacy and education and improving equality and reducing hunger. Current issues in global health include rapidly increasing overweight and obesity – a developed and developing world challenge, alongside the persistence of childhood malnutrition. There is still a high rate of childhood mortality worldwide. Areas of focus include the transmission of infectious diseases including HIV.

Today's global health challenges include the rapidly increasing prevalence of overweight and obesity, which is a challenge for both the developed and developing world (World Obesity Federation 2020). Concurrently, the problem of childhood malnutrition persists, with a high rate of childhood mortality worldwide. It is estimated that malnutrition plays a role in almost half of the cases of under-five child deaths (UN IGME 2018). The transmission of infectious diseases, including HIV, TB, malaria and new airborne diseases, remains a critical challenge for human health and development, with direct consequences for nutritional status. Amongst these challenges is the question of food security and attempts to ensure that every person has enough to eat, of sufficient quality and quantity not just to prevent malnutrition and illness but also to promote good health and well-being. Associated with all these challenges is the need to promote economic development, eliminate poverty and to encourage economic participation, reduction of poor health and improvements in quality of life. Another global health challenge is to promote improvements in literacy and education.

If health is considered as a resource for living as defined by Huber et al. (2011), then this principle is captured by the SDGs. Black et al. (2020) have developed a framework (Figure 1.1) for public health work during the SDG era which places emphasis on children thriving, instead of basic survival, as a means to sustain gains in human development.

Despite these remaining challenges, there have been substantial improvements in human health over the last century. Life expectancy has improved dramatically in past few decades – increasing by 5.5 years across the world between 2000 and 2016 (WHO Global Health Observatory). Some of the reasons cited for this improvement include a reduction in childhood mortality and an increase in access to medications such as antiretrovirals. As life expectancy has increased and younger populations have remained fertile, the world population has nearly doubled since 1960, to reach approximately 7.5 billion people. Just over half of the world population now lives in urban areas (FAO 2019).

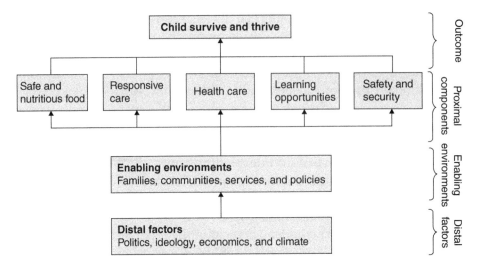

Figure 1.1: Conceptual framework of children surviving and thriving (Black et al. 2020/available by CC BY 4.0 license).

Considering this trend in life expectancy and human population, important challenges for the twenty-first century will be ensuring that all people have enough to eat, and that producing enough food to feed the world population is sustainable. These issues are reflected in SDGs 11 and 12 – sustainable cities and communities, and responsible consumption and production.

Globally, there have been significant reductions in stunting and wasting, but global targets for 2025 and 2030 look unlikely to be met. Sub-Saharan Africa (SSA) and South East Asia have the highest prevalence of undernutrition. The number of those affected in SSA rose from 195 million affected in 2014 to 237 million in 2017.

UN targets for 2030 include to end hunger and ensure food access by all people all year round, and end all forms of malnutrition and ensure sustainable food systems. The forms of malnutrition are discussed throughout this book, with a focus on the manifestations of under- and overnutrition.

Undernutrition and obesity occur together in developing regions, and the phenomenon is called the double burden of malnutrition. A feature of the double burden of malnutrition is a high prevalence of childhood malnutrition with a concurrent high prevalence of adult overweight and obesity. The developmental origins of health and disease hypothesis or metabolic programming is fundamental to understanding the double burden of disease. Exposure to undernutrition during the first thousand days (which includes gestation) of life is associated with permanent metabolic abnormalities that increase the risk of cardiovascular disease.

This phenomenon is also known as the Barker hypothesis. Evidence for the Barker hypothesis emerged during the twentieth century. Analysis of data taken from cohorts of people born during the Dutch famine during World War 2 revealed that people who were exposed to undernutrition during gestation – people whose mothers were undernourished while they were pregnant – are at a higher risk of heart disease in adulthood. Similar results have been observed from the Chinese famine which took place in the 1960s.

Drivers of hunger include economic and political turbulence, armed conflicts and natural disasters. More than 700 million people live in extreme poverty worldwide, approximately 10% of the global population. Many of these people surviving on less than £1.54 a day live in sub-Saharan Africa. Extreme poverty disproportionately affects women. Women between the ages of 25–34 years are more likely to live in extreme poverty than men from this age group. Approximately 20% of children live in extreme poverty, compared with 10% of the global population. The rate of poverty is three times greater in rural areas as compared with urban areas. Approximately 840 million people do not have access to electricity. Energy poverty limits the ability of individuals to store food. Climate change also disproportionately affects people living in low- and middle-income countries. The livelihoods of people in lower socio-economic brackets are more directly related to natural resources. Agriculture remains the main source of income for 40% of the world's population, and small-holder and subsistence farming is more common in low- and middle-income countries. Drivers of food crises in developing countries are exacerbated by climate change (FAO, IFAD, UNICEF, WFP and WHO 2019). Crop diversity has decreased by 75% since 1900. This loss of biodiversity and dietary diversity has resulted in an increased susceptibility to diseases and adverse environmental conditions.

Armed conflict leads to disrupted agricultural production and population displacement. Conflict resulted in the displacement of 42 000 people in 2015, an increase of 381% from 2010.

Sustainable Development Goal 2 is to end hunger and achieve food security and improved nutrition and promote sustainable agriculture. Under Goal 2, the Zero Hunger challenge aims to achieve 100% access to adequate food all year round. It aims to achieve zero stunted children younger than two years and zero malnutrition in pregnancy and early childhood. It aims to make all food systems sustainable as well as achieve 100% growth in small-hold farm productivity and income, especially for women. It aims to achieve zero loss or waste of food. It aims for nutritional supplementation in at-risk groups, including iron, vitamin A and zinc supplementation in children younger than five years.

References

Adams, F. (1849). *Genuine works of Hippocrates*. London: The Sydenham Society.

Black, M.M., Lutter, C.K., and Trude, A.C.B. (2020). All children surviving and thriving: re-envisioning UNICEF's conceptual framework of malnutrition. *Lancet Glob. Health* 8 (6): E766–E767.

Brown, T.M., Cueto, M., and Fee, E. (2006). The World Health Organization and the transition from "international" to "global" public health. *Am. J. Public Health* 96: 62–72. https://doi.org/10.2105/AJPH.2004.050831.

Burr, G.O. and Burr, M.M. (1929). A new deficiency disease produced by the rigid exclusion of fat from the diet. *J. Biol. Chem.* 82 (2): 345–367.

FAO (2019). *The State of Food and Agriculture 2019: Moving forward on food loss and waste reduction*. Rome: Food and Agriculture Organisation.

FAO, IFAD, UNICEF, WFP and WHO (2019). *The State of Food Security and Nutrition in the World 2019*. Rome, FAO: *Safeguarding against economic slow-downs and downturns*.

Gopalan, C. and Rao, K.S.J. (1984). Classifications of undernutrition – their limitations and fallacies. *J. Trop. Paediatr.* 30 (1): 7–10.

Huber, M., Knottnerus, A., Green, L. et al. (2011). How should we define health? *Br. Med. J.* 2011 (343): d4163. https://doi.org/10.1136/bmj.d4163.

Keys, A. (1990). Recollections of pioneers in nutrition: from starvation to cholesterol. *J. Am. Coll. Nutr.* 9 (4): 288–291.

Loewenson, R., Villar, E., Baru, R., and Marten, R. (2021). Engaging globally with how to achieve healthy societies: Insights from India, Latin America and East and Southern Africa. *BMJ Glob. HealthBMJ Global Health* 6 (4): e005257.

Mozaffarian, D., Rosenberg, I., and Uauy, R. (2018). History of modern nutrition science- implications for current research, dietary guidelines, and food policy. *Br. Med. J.* 361: k2392.

Nightingale, F. (1859). *Notes on Nursing*. London, Harrison.

Raven, P.H. and Wagner, D.L. (2021). Agricultural intensification and climate change are rapidly decreasing insect biodiversity. *PNAS* 118 (2): e2002548117. http://dx.doi.org/10.1073/pnas.2002548117.

Skiadas, P.K. and Lascaratos, J.G. (2001). Dietetics in ancient Greek philosophy: Plato's concepts on healthy diet. *Eur. J. Clin. Nutr.Eur J Clin Nutr* 55 (7): 532–537.

Trowell, H.C. and Davies, J.N.P. (1952). Kwashiorkor: Nutritional background, history, distribution and incidence. *Br. Med. J.* 2 (4788): 796–798.

UN IGME (2018). *Levels and trends in child mortality: Report 2018. Estimates developed by the UN Inter-agency Group for Child Mortality Estimation*. New York: United Nations Children's Fund.

WHO (1948). *Constitution of the World Health Organisation*. Geneva: World Health Organisation.

WHO (1987). *Ottawa Charter for Health Promotion*. Ottawa, ON: World Health Organisation.

World Obesity Federation (2020). *Obesity: Missing the 2025 global targets*. London: World Obesity Federation.

2 Assessing Nutritional Status

2.1 Introduction

Nutrition assessment is made up of four components: anthropometry, the measurement of body dimensions and morphology; biochemistry that gives an indication of the body's interaction with nutrients; clinical assessment that evaluates the physical manifestations of nutritional intake; and dietary assessment that estimates nutritional intake in the form of food and nutrients (Patterson and Pietinen 2004). Gibson (2005) defines nutrition assessment as 'the interpretation of information from dietary, laboratory, anthropometric and clinical studies'.

Useful indicators for nutrition assessment need to be valid and reliable – they must be capable of measuring the outcome they intend to measure with accuracy, and the results must be repeatable. Ideally, measures will be the same for individuals and populations. This allows for easier comparison, as well as enhanced familiarity with indicators across different sectors such as surveillance and clinical work. They should be minimally invasive. Good measurements should be inexpensive, particularly if they are to be used in large field studies or to screen large groups of people. Finally, measurements should be easy to collect and interpret. This helps to increase the likelihood of measurements being taken appropriately and reduces the risk of errors in the collection and interpretation of data.

Anthropometric measurements assess body composition and morphology and are a useful component of nutrition assessment.

2.2 Measuring Weight and Height in Infants and Young Children

Nutritional status is most commonly assessed using anthropometric indicators. This section outlines gold standard techniques for measuring weight using scales, length using an infantometer and height using a stadiometer.

Nutrition and Global Health, First Edition. Shawn W. McLaren.
© 2023 John Wiley & Sons Ltd. Published 2023 by John Wiley & Sons Ltd.

Anthropometry is the most universally applicable, non-invasive method of assessing growth in children (De Onis 2015). The WHO Child Growth Standards represent normal growth under optimal environmental conditions and can be used to assess children everywhere, regardless of ethnicity, socio-economic status and type of feeding (De Onis et al. 2006).

2.2.1 Measuring Infant Weight

The weight of infants and young children is monitored as a measure of growth. As infants have poor motor control, infant scales are designed with a bucket to measure the infant's weight recumbently. Recumbent weight is an appropriate measurement for children under two years of age (Centre for Disease Control 2007).

In 2006, the WHO revised the international growth reference for infant and under-five child growth. The result was the WHO child growth standard, used globally to assess the nutritional status and growth of children.

The weight of infants and children is assessed using a scale. Weight is interpreted using the WHO standard weight for age (WFA) Z-score chart. This chart is used from birth to five years; thereafter, the WHO reference is used. There are separate charts for boys and girls. The boys' WFA Z-score chart is shown below.

Once the weight is taken, it is compared to the standard for the child's age at the time of measurement. If the WFA is below the −2 line, the child is classified as underweight (Figure 2.1). A weight plotted above

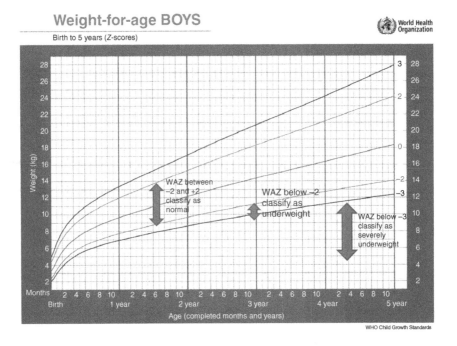

Figure 2.1: Assessing weight using the WHO (2006) growth chart.

Source: WHO Child Growth Standards.

the −2 line is considered normal. The interpretations are included in the growth chart below. Weight should be assessed at every clinic visit for children younger than five years.

1. **Measuring Weight**

   As children get older, they get bigger. One method for deciding whether a child is growing well is to check their weight, as a child growing will also grow heavier. The child's weight can then be compared to the expected weight for their age, which is most often done using the WFA Growth Chart.

Weighing infants:

Step 1: Calibrate the scale to ensure that the weight reading is accurate. Test the accuracy of the scale by weighing an object with a known weight (for example, a 1 kg packet of sugar). If the weight displayed is incorrect, calibrate the scale.

Step 2: Ask the infant's mother or caregiver to remove the infant's outer clothes (jackets, pants and shoes).

Step 3: Turn the infant scale on and place a clean Chux pad on the scale. Press 'Tare' to 'zero' the scale before placing the infant on the scale.

Step 4: Place the infant on the centre of the scale, lying on his or her back. Allow the weight reading to settle and then record the weight on the WFA Growth Chart in kilograms (kg) to the nearest 0.01 kg (10 g).

Weighing Children:

Step 1: Calibrate the scale to ensure that the weight reading is accurate. Test the accuracy of the scale by weighing an object with a known weight (for example, a 1 kg packet of mealie meal). If the weight displayed is incorrect, calibrate the scale.

Step 2: Ask the child's mother or caregiver to remove the child's outer clothes (jackets, pants and shoes).

Step 3: Put the child on the standing scale, allow the weight reading to settle and then record the weight on the WFA Growth Chart in kilograms (kg) to the nearest 0.01 kg (10 g).

2.2.2 Measuring Infant Length

Length is measured using an infantometer. Fixed infantometers with a movable foot piece are often used in clinics and hospitals, while a foldable portable infantometer is employed in community settings such as growth monitoring sites, health posts and during community health worker visits to homes or crèches. Length is recorded in centimetres (cm) to the nearest 0.1 cm (1 mm).

Parallax is the phenomenon that occurs when observers of measurements record an erroneous measurement due to incorrect viewing angles. This is avoided (and the accuracy of measurements improved) by assessing measurements at eye level.

Weight changes constantly, but children grow in length or height more gradually. Measuring length refers to infants who are too young to stand unassisted, and height refers to how tall a child is when they are able to stand on their own (at around 24 months old). Length is measured using an infantometer or length board, as described below. Height may be assessed using a stadiometer or graduated vertical height stick.

Length and height are very important indicators of growth in children. This process requires two people (a 'recorder' and an 'examiner') for accuracy and involves the caretaker or parent to ensure that the baby feels safe and comfortable. Length is measured using an infantometer (length board or foldable length mat).

Measuring infants:

Step 1: Remove the infant's outer clothes, undo braided hairstyles, and place a clean Chux pad on the infantometer length board.

Step 2: The child must be positioned with the feet oriented towards the movable foot piece, and the head resting against the stationary head piece. One researcher supports the head and records the measurement while the other positions the feet and examines the length measurement. Infants may become agitated (irritable and crying) in a recumbent (lying) and vulnerable position, so it is advised that the infant's caretaker position her or himself between the recorder and examiner.

Step 3: The infant's back and legs must be straight, with the sole of the foot at a right angle to the length board for a reading to be accurate. Extremely uncomfortable children may be recorded with only one straight leg. A gentle stroke along the inside of the infant's foot may help to get it into the correct position.

Step 4: Shift the foot piece up against the infants' feet and take the measurement. Record the length on the Length/Height for Age Growth Chart, in centimetres (cm) to the nearest 0.1 cm (1 mm).

Measuring Children:

Children who can stand can be measured using a stadiometer (adjustable height stick):

Step 1: Remove the child's shoes and head dress (hats and braided hairstyles).

Step 2: The child needs to stand with his or her back to the height stick. The heels of the feet, bum, back and head must touch the height stick.

Step 3: While the child breathes in, gently lower the horizontal sliding piece onto the top of the child's head. Read and record the height in centimetres (cm), to the nearest 0.1 cm (1 mm) in the Height for Age Growth Chart in the RTHB.

Length and height are interpreted using the WHO standard length for age (LFA) chart, as shown below. The length of the child, measured in centimetres, is plotted against the age of the child at the time of measurement. If the plotted point is below the −2 line, the child is classified as stunted. If the LFA is below the −3 line, the child is severely stunted.

2.2.3 Mid-Upper Arm Circumference Tapes

Non-stretch measuring tapes are made specifically for measuring mid-upper arm circumference (MUAC). The MUAC is recorded to the nearest 0.1 cm (1 mm).

Precautions should be taken to reduce the risk of parallax error when measuring MUAC. All measurements should be consistently performed on the left-hand side of the body, unless a confounding factor such as an amputation or cast makes this impossible. All measurements were recorded to the nearest 1 mm.

2.2.3.1 Mid-Upper Arm Circumference

MUAC is assessed using a flexible tape measure. It is a measurement of the amount of bone, muscle, fat and skin on the arm. MUAC may be used as an indirect method to assess the degree of wasting of fat and muscle stores in infants and young children. Weight for length is the gold standard but many fieldworkers in EC do not measure it because they have no access to scales. MUAC is a cheap, simple and effective alternative.

An MUAC measurement of less than 11.5 cm is classified as severe acute malnutrition (SAM). A measurement that is between 11.5 and 12.5 cm is classified as moderate acute malnutrition (MAM). An MUAC of greater than 12.5 cm is considered not acutely malnourished. Children younger than five years should have their MUAC assessed every three months.

The measuring technique for MUAC begins with finding the acromion process on the shoulder. The left arm should be measured. The arm should be bent at the elbow with the palm open and facing upwards. The measuring tape should be placed on the back of the arm

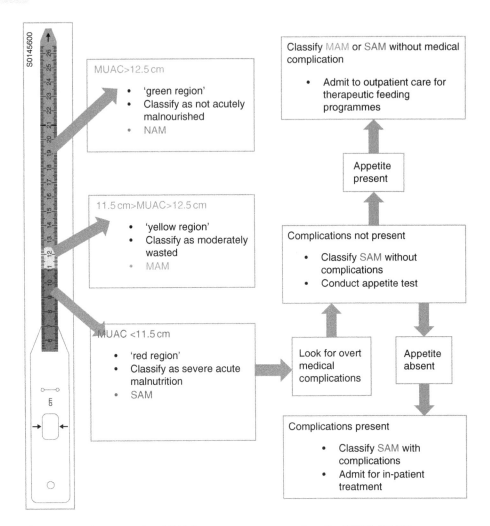

Figure 2.2: Interpreting MUAC measurements using the WHO (2013) recommendations.

and the distance between the acromion process and elbow measured. This measurement should be halved, and this midpoint marked on the arm with a suitable pencil or pen as the mid-upper arm. The MUAC tape should then be placed horizontally at this point, allowing the circumference of the arm to be measured. The measuring tape should make contact with the arm all the way around, but should not be so tight as to compress the arm. The interpretation of MUAC is given in the diagram presented in Figure 2.2.

2.2.3.1.1 Measuring Mid-Upper Arm Circumference MUAC is also measured using a non-stretchable measuring tape. MUAC is an extremely easy and reliable tool for diagnosing SAM and MAM.

Step 1: Begin standing on the right-hand side of the infant or young child, the infant's weight evenly distributed, shoulders relaxed and right arm hanging freely at the side.

Step 2: Find the acromion process at the end of the shoulder and mark it with a cosmetic pen. From this point, place a tape measure along the length of the upper arm to find the numerical midpoint. Mark this point with the cosmetic pen.

Step 3: Move the infant's arm into a position where it is bent perpendicularly at the elbow, palm facing upwards. Measure the circumference around the infant's arm at the marked midpoint and record to the nearest 0.1 cm (1 mm).

The use of the current MUAC guidelines is given in the diagram shown in Figure 2.2.

2.3 Growth References and Growth Standards

The NCHS growth reference was developed by the Ohio Fels Research Institute during the 1970s, providing healthcare workers with a yardstick to measure infant growth against. Later, the use of these growth reference charts outside of the United States was questioned as the dynamics of infant growth became more apparent. This led to the development of the WHO (2006) growth standards, which have been adopted by many countries across the world.

Prior to the introduction of the WHO (2006) Child Growth Standards as a growth reference, the majority of countries used the NCHS/WHO growth reference, with some opting for CDC 2000 or a local growth reference (de Onis et al. 2012). The interpretation of infant growth trajectory is highly dependent on the growth reference used (de Onis 2015). The NCHS/WHO growth reference was developed from longitudinal data collected by the Ohio Fels Research Institute prior to 1975 (Dibley et al. 1987). It also made use of cross-sectional data from the US Health Examination Surveys from 1960 to 1975. The international use of the NCHS/WHO growth reference was later in question, as it did not include infants and young children from a diverse range of socio-economic backgrounds or geographic locations (De Onis et al. 2004a,b). This fact raised concerns that the growth reference would not be applicable to children living outside of the United States of America. The sample was predominantly formula-fed, which also meant that the growth reference might not accurately represent the growth of breast-fed infants (De

Onis et al. 2004a,b). Further methodological criticisms were raised because samples for the NCHS reference were obtained from children at three-month intervals and fitted to a curve. This method did not accurately represent the rapid and dynamic growth of infants during the first year of life (Cloete et al. 2013). The difference in growth trajectory between the formula-fed infant and the breast-fed infant is pronounced, and the most significant differences are observed between the youngest infants (Martorell and Young 2012). The anthropometries of breast-fed and formula-fed infants during the first months of life differ significantly (Alvarez-Uria et al. 2012). Initially, breast-fed infants are heavier and taller than formula-fed infants (Duggan 2013). Breast-fed infants then become lighter than formula-fed infants after two months of age (Alvarez-Uria et al. 2012) but retain their greater height (Duggan 2013). This means that the breast-fed infant has a lower WFH than the formula-fed infant and is identified as acutely malnourished at a higher WFH than the formula-fed infant (Duggan 2013).

These problems with growth reference led to the development of WHO (2006) growth Standard (De Onis and the WHO Multicentre Growth Reference Study Group 2012). The WHO (2006) growth Standard included infants and young children from a diverse set of social, cultural and national backgrounds and described the growth trajectory of the breast-fed infant (De Onis 2015). The WHO (2006) Growth Standard differed from the other growth references available in that it was purposely designed to produce a standard. This was achieved by selecting healthy children living under conditions likely to favour the achievement of their full genetic growth potential. Mothers of the children selected for the construction of the standards engaged in fundamental health-promoting practices, including practicing exclusive breastfeeding and not smoking. The study design for the WHO (2006) growth standard included shorter measurement intervals, resulting in a better tool for monitoring the rapid and changing rate of growth in early infancy (De Onis et al. 2007).

The differences in growth trajectory translate to large differences in the estimated prevalence of wasting and stunting when the NCHS/WHO growth reference is compared with the WHO (2006) Growth Standard. Using the Growth Standard revealed a higher prevalence of stunting amongst infants younger than 12 months when compared with the Growth Reference (Martorell and Young 2012). This difference in prevalence estimates was even more prominent amongst younger infants less than six months old. The estimated prevalence of wasting and stunting tripled using the WHO (2006) Growth Standard compared with the NCHS/WHO Growth reference (Martorell and Young 2012).

The advantage of the WHO (2006) Growth Standard is that younger and therefore more vulnerable children are more likely to be identified as malnourished.

Similar limitations apply to the CDC 2000 growth reference. The CDC 2000 growth reference included both formula and breast-fed infants and children. The CDC 2000 child is typically heavier and shorter than the WHO (2006) Growth Standard child (De Onis et al. 2007). Healthy breast-fed infants track along the WHO standard's weight-for-age mean Z-score while appearing to falter on the CDC chart from two months onwards. The differences in prevalence of malnutrition in infants and young children are affected by the differences in the WHO (2006) Growth Standard and CDC 2000 growth reference in a slightly different manner to the WHO (2006) Growth Standard compared with the NCHS/WHO growth standard. WHO (2006) Growth Standard reveals lower rates of undernutrition amongst infants younger than six months while simultaneously identifying higher rates of overweight and obesity (De Onis et al. 2007).

2.3.1 The WHO (2006) Growth Standard Charts

The majority of countries were relying on WFA as the sole nutritional indicator prior to the introduction of the WHO Child Growth Standards in 2006 (De Onis et al. 2004a,b). Height for age (HFA) was being used by only 41% of countries and 23% were monitoring WFL as part of their growth monitoring and promotion activities (De Onis et al. 2004a,b). This was problematic as WFA on its own is not sufficient to identify the range of manifestations of childhood malnutrition that includes stunting, wasting and overweight (Semba and Bloem 2008). After the introduction of the WHO child growth standards, WFA was still the most universally adopted growth indicator, but the gap between the use of WFA and other anthropometric indicators of child growth had become smaller (de Onis et al. 2012). By 2011, HFA was used by 83% of countries and WFL by 70% of countries (de Onis et al. 2012).

2.3.1.1 Calculating Z-Scores

The WHO has used the following equation to calculate Z-scores or standard deviations:

$$Z-\text{score} = \frac{\text{Observed value} - \text{median value of the reference population}}{\text{Standard deviation value of the reference population}}$$

The *Z*-scores describe an even distribution around the median or reference *Z*-score (0) in a similar manner to standard deviations (SD), and the two terms are often used interchangeably. *Z*-scores offer several advantages for interpreting child growth. *Z*-scores have a linear scale, meaning that there is a fixed interval between *Z*-scores for children of a specific age. This means that the interval in centimetres between the 0 and +1 *Z*-score is the same interval between the +1 and +2 *Z*-scores on the same distribution. Results of anthropometric measurements are comparable across age groups when using the *Z*-scores as they have the same statistical relation to their distribution around the reference at all ages. The *Z*-scores are sex-independent, therefore a given *Z*-score for a male child is comparable to the same *Z*-score value for a female child. These characteristics of *Z*-score distributions allow researchers to combine data from different age groups and sexes to produce summary statistics for populations such as means, standard deviations or standard errors.

2.3.2 Weight for Age *Z*-Score Growth Chart

WFA is an indicator of body weight at the time of measurement in relation to the age of the child. An example of the WHO (2006) WFA growth chart is given in Figure 2.3. A WFA of more than two SD below the median of the WHO (2006) Growth Standard is considered underweight for age. A WFA below three SD of the WHO (2006) Growth Standard is classified as severely underweight for age (WHO 2008). WFA may be used to identify underweight in children, but it is not used for identifying overweight and obesity (WHO 2008).

2.3.3 Height for Age *Z*-Score Growth Chart

Linear growth is assessed by measuring the length or height of an infant or child and comparing the measurements with a standard for the same age and sex (Figure 2.4). The conventional definition of moderate stunting is length or height for age below −2 standard deviations (SD) from the median of the WHO (2006) Growth Standard (WHO 2008). Severely stunted children have HFA below −3 SD of the median.

2.3.4 Weight for Height *Z*-Score Growth Chart

Weight for height is a measure of body weight in relation to attained linear growth (WHO 2008). This nutritional screening method is independent of age, eliminating challenges such as accurately estimating a child's age (Hall et al. 2011).

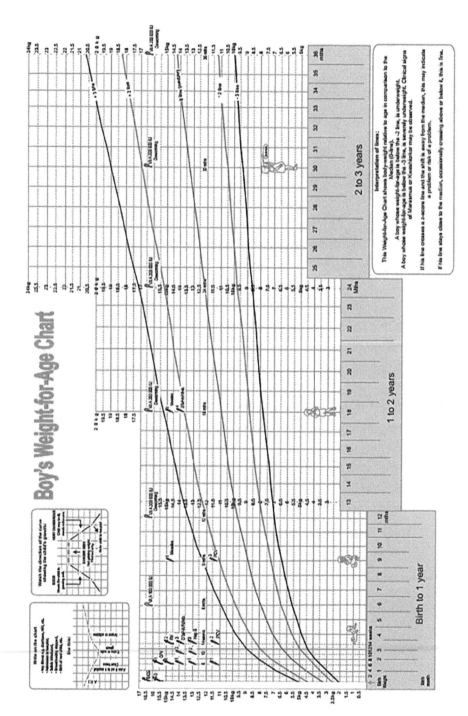

Figure 2.3: The WHO (2006) weight for age growth chart.

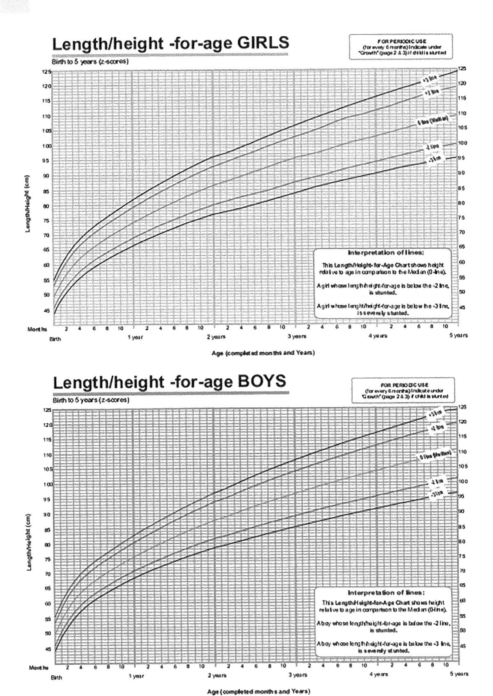

Figure 2.4: The WHO (2006) height for age growth chart.

The weight for height growth chart is used to assess wasting in infants and children (Figure 2.5). A weight for height Z-score of below -3 SD from the median of the WHO (2006) growth standard is defined as SAM, and a WFH Z-score between -2 and -3 SD from the median is defined as MAM (WHO and UNICEF 2009). WHZ greater than 2 SD above the median is commonly used as a cut-off value for overweight amongst children, and WHZ above 3 SD higher than the median is defined as obese (Thomas et al. 2016; Retamal and Nicholas Mascie-Taylor 2019).

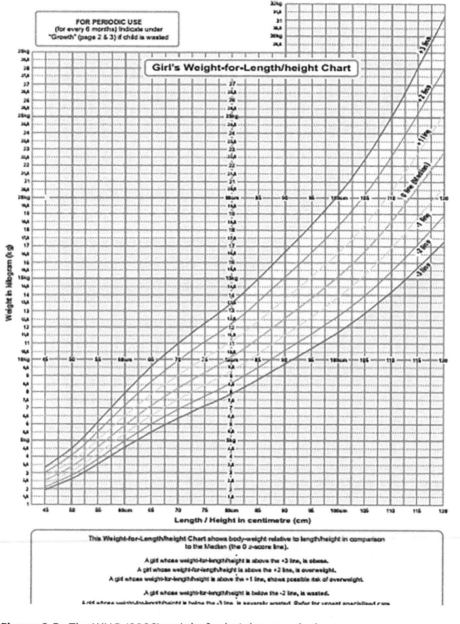

Figure 2.5: The WHO (2006) weight for height growth chart.

Source: Vasundhara et al. 2020/John Wiley & Sons/CC BY 4.0.

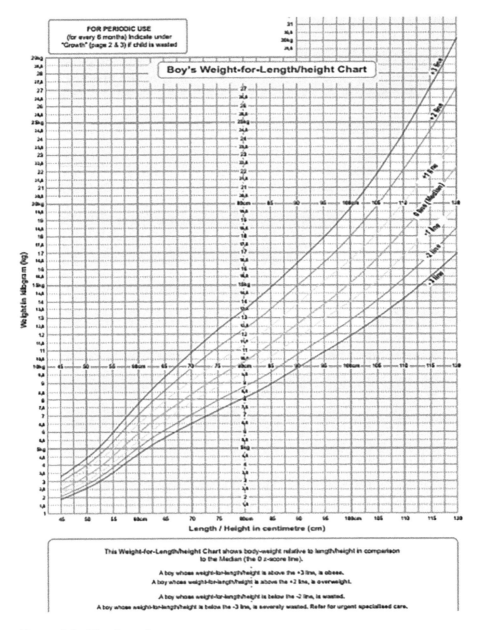

Figure 2.5: (Continued)

2.3.5 BMI for Age Z-Score Growth Chart

The WHO has developed a body mass index (BMI) for age growth charts for the WHO (2006) Growth Standard. The International Obesity Task Force (IOTF) has also produced cut-off values for interpreting BMI for age in children, which is often used in evaluating overweight and obesity in children and adolescents (Cole and Lobstein 2012). Both the WHO

(2006) Growth Standard and IOTF BMI for age can be used to identify individuals as underweight, normal weight, overweight or obese.

BMI-for-age requires the fieldworker to calculate the BMI of the child before plotting on the growth chart. The equation for BMI is

$$\text{BMI}\left(\text{kg}\,/\,\text{m}^2\right) = \frac{\text{Weight}\left(\text{kg}\right)}{\text{Height}^2\left(\text{cm}\right)}$$

2.4 Plotting and Interpreting the Growth Chart

This section outlines the method for plotting and interpreting the WHO (2006) growth standard charts. The WHO has produced growth charts for weight-for-age, height-for-age, weight-for-height and BMI-for-age. Each chart is associated with specific conditions resulting from under- and over-nutrition.

2.4.1 Weight-for-Age

Weight-for-age will tell you whether a child is underweight or not. It has the advantage of providing a weight 'history' of the child as the weights are plotted over time. Additionally, by regular monitoring, it can be used to catch growth faltering before the problem becomes clinical.

To start, you will need to obtain the child's weight in kilograms and age in months. As the WHO (2006) growth standard charts are sex-specific, you will need to ensure that you have the correct chart for a male or female child. The child's age is plotted along the x-axis (horizontal) of the growth chart and the weight is plotted along the y-axis (vertical). The child's WFA at the time of measurement is the point where the coordinates of age and weight meet by drawing a vertical line upwards from the x-axis at the child's current age and a horizontal line across the chart from the y-axis at the child's current weight.

The position of the point plotted is interpreted in relation to the Z-score lines on the growth chart. Interpretations are given in Table 2.1. The line labelled '0' is the median line. This is the median weight for a child of that age.

2.4.2 Height-for-Age

Height for age is used to determine whether a child is stunted or at risk of stunting and, like weight-for-age, provides a linear history of the child's height attainment. The method for obtaining the height for age is the

Table 2.1: Interpretation of the weight for age growth chart.

Position on growth chart	Interpretation
WAZ > +3	Possibly overweight: confirm with WFL Z-score
WAZ > +2	
−1 > WAZ > +2	Normal weight (growing well)
−1 > WAZ > −2	Mildly underweight
WAZ < −2	Moderately underweight
WAZ < −3	Severely underweight

Table 2.2: Interpreting the length and height for age growth chart.

Position on growth chart	Interpretation
Above the +2 line	Normal height (growing well)
Between the +2 and −1 lines	
Between −1 and −2 lines	Mildly stunted
Below the −2 line	Moderately stunted
Below the −3 line	Severely stunted

same as for weight for height. You will need to obtain the child's age in months and height in centimetres.

On the height-for-age growth chart, age is plotted along the x-axis (horizontal) and height is plotted along the y-axis (vertical). Once the child's height and age have been obtained, these values can be used to determine the child's height for age using the growth chart. The WHO (2006) growth standard charts are sex specific, so you will need to use the correct chart for the child's sex. The interpretation of the length and height for the age growth chart is presented in Table 2.2.

The weight for height growth chart provides an interpretation of the child's weight in relation to their attained height or length. This growth chart is used to identify moderate and severe acute malnutrition, as well as overweight and obesity. This index of growth does not make the use of the child's age and therefore does not 'tell a story' of the child's growth trajectory over time. This has a practical advantage in the field as the exact date of birth or age of the child is not necessary to interpret the growth chart. Interpretations of this growth chart are given in Table 2.3.

Table 2.3: Interpreting the weight-for-height growth chart.

Position on growth chart	Interpretation
Above +2 line	Overweight
Between +2 and −1 lines	Normal weight for height (growing well; or both stunted and underweight at the same time)
Between −1 and −2 lines	Mild acute malnutrition
Below −2 line	Moderate acute malnutrition
Below −3 line	Severe acute malnutrition

2.5 Mid-Upper Arm Circumference

MUAC is a simple measurement that is used widely by aid agencies to screen children for malnutrition. It is also the subject of furious debate in the scientific community as its ability to identify malnourished children appears to be region specific. This section outlines the technique for measuring MUAC, its interpretation and its applications in the field.

MUAC measures the circumference of the arm including bone, muscle, adipose and dermal tissues. The MUAC may therefore be used as an indirect method to assess the degree of wasting of fat and muscle stores in infants and young children (Briend et al. 2015).

The simplicity of MUAC makes it an ideal diagnostic tool for identifying malnutrition (Briend et al. 2015). The MUAC can be measured easily, and has been shown to be well understood by health workers and children's caregivers (Blackwell et al. 2015) and is able to accurately identify malnutrition even with extremely limited training (Blackwell et al. 2015). These factors allow for MUAC to be measured more frequently than WHZ. According to Briend and Zimicki (1986), MUAC should be measured monthly for optimal monitoring of nutritional status, which is more achievable than WHZ. The increased frequency of MUAC measurement aids in earlier identification of SAM, which may help in reducing the time between the beginning of malnutrition and the onset of complications (Briend et al. 2015).

However, there are growing concerns about the current MUAC cut-off values for identifying infants and young children with MAM and SAM. One concern is that such low cut-off values mean that children are extremely malnourished before they reach the threshold for intervention (Joseph et al. 2002). Although there is sufficient evidence that WHZ Z- scores and MUAC may be used as independent criteria for identifying cases of high-risk malnutrition (Briend and Prinzo 2009), Laillou et al.

(2014) found that the WHO-recommended MUAC cut-off values identified a significantly different set of young children as malnourished when compared with WHZ Z-scores. Ali et al. (2013) recognised that there was little overlap between the groups of children identified by either MUAC or WHZ Z-score as severely malnourished. It has been estimated that there is an overlap of 40% between WHZ and MUAC (WHO and UNICEF 2009). However, in spite of the lack of overlap, their investigation in Bangladesh led these researchers to conclude that using MUAC alone is acceptable to identify SAM in children. Based on their results, Ali et al. (2013) recommend that a higher MUAC cut-off value might increase the number of children included in nutrition interventions, who are at a high risk of nutritional deterioration.

There has also been some concern regarding the use of a single MUAC cut-off value for children aged between 6 and 59 months. De Onis et al. (1997) showed that MUAC is in fact age-dependent. It was found that older children within this age group tend to have higher mid-upper arm circumferences than younger children. This in turn leads to an under-diagnosis of wasting in older children and more diagnoses of wasting amongst younger children (De Onis et al. 1997). Furthermore, the risk of mortality decreases as age increases, making MUAC's ability to predict mortality risk biased towards younger children and not necessarily descriptive of mortality risk for the whole age group (De Onis et al. 1997).

Dairo et al. (2012) found that MUAC has poor sensitivity in identifying wasting in children younger than two years using current cut-off values. However, Burden et al. (2001) found that MUAC was a reliable tool for identifying malnourished patients when compared with other markers of malnutrition ($p < 0.05$).

2.6 Assessing Adults: Waist Circumference and BMI

The most common method to assess adult nutritional status is by using BMI. This method is frequently used to assess both individuals and populations. This section outlines the method of measuring weight and height and calculating BMI in adults. It also offers alternative measures, including waist and hip circumference, and how these are measured, interpreted and applied.

2.6.1 Body Mass Index

BMI, as an index of weight and height, does not differentiate between the tissues that the height and weight are composed of such as skeletal mass, muscle or adipose tissue (McCarthy 2014; Romero-Corral et al. 2006). BMI does not identify where fat is distributed, which is also an important determinant of cardiovascular disease risk (McCarthy 2014). Obese adults differ in the amount of excess fat stored as well as the distribution of the fat within the body (Garrow 1988). The distribution of fat affects the disease risks that result from obesity (Courtinhop et al. 2011). In subjects with coronary artery disease (CAD), including those with normal and high BMI, central obesity but not BMI is directly associated with mortality (Courtinhop et al. 2011). There is some evidence that measuring waist circumference is comparable in estimating hypertension risk as BMI amongst adults and has the advantage of specifically identifying central obesity (Ononamadu et al. 2017).

2.6.2 Waist Circumference, Waist-to-Hip Ratio and Waist-to-Height Ratio

Waist circumference is a simple measure for identifying overweight and obese individuals for intervention (Lean et al. 1995). Cut-off values for overweight (94 cm for men and 80 cm for women) and obesity (102 cm for mean and 88 cm for women) are both sufficiently sensitive and specific to identify overweight and obese individuals (Lean et al. 1995). The limitations of BMI have been discussed previously. Waist circumference has shown to be a significant predictor of obesity-related co-morbidities (Janssen et al. 2004). Measures of central obesity are better at predicting cardiovascular disease risk than BMI (Huxley et al. 2010). Another anthropometric indicator using waist circumference is waist-to-height ratio (WHR). WHR identifies people at higher risk of cardiovascular disease than a matrix made from BMI and waist circumference (Ashwell and Gibson 2016). Individuals with a WHR greater than 0.5 but a healthy ($18.5–24.9\,\text{kg/m}^2$) BMI had more cardiometabolic risk factors than those with a WHR less than 0.5 and healthy BMI (Ashwell and Gibson 2016). This suggests that WHR is an early indicator of health risk, before BMI is out of the healthy range. The WHO (2008) has suggested that waist circumference and waist-to-hip ratio have potential uses for nutritional surveillance activities as well as for screening. Beyond screening, these anthropometric indicators can be used for diagnosis and clinical decisions to treat in individuals and in assessing community intervention (WHO 2008).

2.6.2.1 Assessing Nutritional Status During Pregnancy

Nutritional status amongst pregnant women has been identified as an important determinant of pregnancy outcomes. Therefore, assessing nutritional status during pregnancy is important. There are a few

Table 2.4: Institute of Medicine weight gains during pregnancy according to pre-pregnancy BMI.

BMI	Classification	Weight gain
<18.5 kg/m²	Underweight	12.5–18 kg
18.5–24.9 kg/m²	Normal weight	11.5–16 kg
25–29.9 kg/m²	Overweight	7–11.5 kg
>30 kg/m²	Obese	5–9 kg

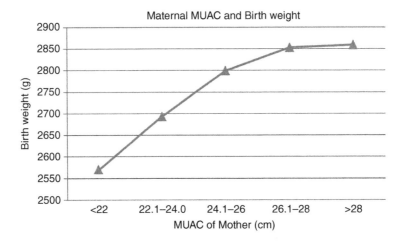

Figure 2.6: Relationship between maternal MUAC and infant birth weight Vasundhara et al 2020 / John Wiley & Sons / CC BY 4.0.

anthropometric measures available which can identify the risk of under- or over-nutrition during pregnancy. These include BMI, mid-upper arm circumference and weight gain or changes in weight.

The Institute of Medicine has proposed weight gain ranges based on pre-pregnancy BMI. These are presented in Table 2.4. Women who are overweight at the point of conception benefit from less weight gain during pregnancy, while those who are classified as underweight have a higher healthy weight gain during pregnancy.

Mid-upper arm circumference may be a useful indicator of nutritional status during gestation Figure 2.6. This is because a relationship has been observed between maternal MUAC and infant birth weight (Vasundhara et al. 2020). Therefore, birth weight of the infant, an important predictor for birth outcomes, can be predicted by maternal MUAC. Cut-off values for MUAC in pregnancy need to be population-specific and these cut-off values should be based on cost–benefit analyses specific to the population and health system they are used in (Vasundhara et al. 2020).

2.7 Biochemical Indicators of Nutritional Status

This section describes the blood tests taken to test common micronutrient deficiencies, including serum retinol for vitamin A status, haemoglobin and ferritin for iron status and indicators of chronic diseases of lifestyle including serum cholesterol and HbA1c.

Biochemical assessment contributes to the overall nutritional assessment and is used to detect subclinical nutrient deficiency states and to confirm clinical diagnoses. The biochemical tests supplement other methods of nutritional assessment to provide a more complete and clearer picture of the nutritional status of an individual or population. The result of the laboratory test is compared against a reference range to determine whether an individual is deficient in a nutrient. Laboratory tests can be static tests or functional tests. Static biochemical tests measure concentrations of nutrients in biological fluids tissues, or the urinary excretion rate of a nutrient or its metabolites (Gibson 2005). Functional tests assess changes in the activities of enzymes that depend on a specific nutrient or the concentration of specific blood components that are dependent on a nutrient.

2.7.1 Limitations of Biochemical Tests

Factors will affect the reliability of biochemical tests. It is important to note that serum concentrations of nutrients can vary depending on absorption, genetics and disease states. Dietary intake and timing of exposure to nutrients including recent dietary intake and the effects of dietary manipulation can affect observed values. Inappropriate quality control and sample collection can cause inaccuracies in results (Blanck et al. 2003). The validity, precision, sensitivity and specificity of laboratory tests for identifying nutritional deficiencies and underlying conditions should be considered when interpreting laboratory tests. Validity refers to how well values are measured in relation to the true value. This is sometimes also described as accuracy. Precision refers to the repeatability of the measurement. An inaccurate measurement may still be precise. Sensitivity and specificity are related to interpreting results, and deal with true positives and false negatives. Sensitivity is a measure of a diagnostic tool's ability to identify the presence of a health condition. In other words, it is the tool's ability to correctly identify 'true positives'. The specificity of a diagnostic tool refers to the accuracy of correct diagnoses made by the tool. A sensitive and specific diagnostic test includes as many 'true positives' as possible, while minimising the number of 'false negatives' obtained using the tool.

2.7.2 Iron Markers

Haemoglobin is present in red blood cells. It is made up of four units, and each unit contains a haem group and a globin protein. Each of the four haem groups contains iron as part of its structure, which has a strong affinity for oxygen. The function of haemoglobin is to carry oxygen from the lungs to the tissues of the body.

Myoglobin is the oxygen reserve found in muscle tissue. Muscles have high demands for oxygen. Myoglobin has a similar structure to haemoglobin, except that it is made up of one haem unit and a globin chain.

Ferritin and hemosiderin are two storage proteins for iron. They facilitate a reversible storage of iron and have a large capacity for storing this mineral. Ferritin is more metabolically active than hemosiderin. Transferrin is a transport protein for iron, which is used to transport iron between different sites in the body.

2.7.3 Site of Iron Absorption

Dietary iron is found in two forms – haem and non-haem iron. Haem iron comes from animal sources, whereas non-haem iron comes from plant sources. Both haem and non-haem iron are absorbed in the duodenum. Iron from food sources is usually bound to proteins. Iron is released from carrier proteins as part of the digestive process. Iron enters the gut mucosa cells via active absorption, but there are separate membrane-bound transport proteins for haem and non-haem iron. Haem iron is more readily absorbed than non-haem iron by a factor of two or three, and haem iron absorption is mostly independent of other dietary components. Ferrous iron is extracted from haem by haem oxidase once inside the duodenal cell. Non-haem iron is obtained from plant sources and comes in the form of ferric iron (Fe^{3+}), which is insoluble and poorly absorbed compared to haem iron. An enzyme on the border of the duodenal cell reduces ferric iron to ferrous iron (Fe^{2+}), which can be absorbed more readily. Once ferric iron has been reduced to ferrous iron in the gut lumen, it is absorbed via a membrane protein named divalent metal transporter 1 (DMT-1). Ferrous iron reacts with oxygen to produce reactive oxidative species (ROS) and therefore must be stored safely. Free iron found in the duodenal cell is known as the 'labile iron pool'. Once iron has entered the mucosal cells, it is stored in ferritin until it is required by the body. A small proportion of iron is used in enzymes. Iron that is not stored immediately or used must be transported to the rest of the body for storage and use elsewhere. This process is presented in Figure 2.7.

Transferrin is a transport protein for iron. It makes iron soluble, prevents iron-mediated free radical activity and facilitates the transport of iron into the cells. Transferrin is synthesised in the liver, and most tissues

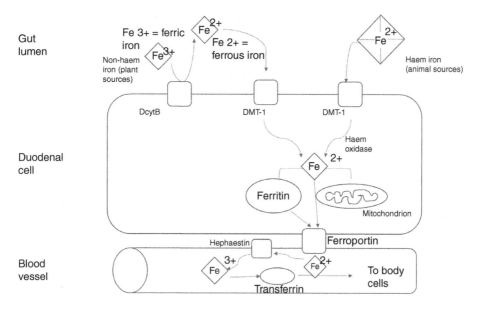

Figure 2.7: Absorption of iron at the site of the duodenal cell.

have transferrin receptors (Ganz 2003). Iron homeostasis is managed at the site of the duodenal cell. The release of iron into the blood for transport is mediated by a membrane-bound protein known as ferroportin. As only ferric iron can be attached to transferrin, a protein called haephesterin reduces the ferrous iron leaving the duodenal cell, converting it to ferric iron for transportation. The liver produces a protein called hepcidin. Hepcidin binds to the ferroportin and haephesterin complex, changing its shape and causing it to be resorbed into the duodenal cell where it is catabolised. Hepcidin is released in response to iron repletion – it prevents too much iron from being absorbed into the blood. However, hepcidin is also released in response to inflammation – this can result in signs of iron deficiency in spite of an adequate diet as a result of acute illness – or even with chronic low-intensity inflammation associated with overweight and obesity.

2.7.4 Identifying the Causes of Anaemia

Anaemia can be caused by nutritional deficiency of iron or by chronic infections. Three related biochemical tests can differentiate the causes for anaemia – namely serum iron, total iron binding capacity and transferrin saturation. Total iron binding capacity is the sum of all unfilled iron-binding sites on transferrin. The quantity of iron saturating all iron binding sites on transferrin is measured after exogenous iron is added to serum. The test identifies that iron deficiency is the number of free iron binding sites as transferrin increases (Ganz 2003).

Ferritin is one of the storage proteins for iron. Serum concentration of ferritin corresponds with the amount of iron that is stored. Serum ferritin concentration reflects iron deficiency, excess iron or normal iron stores and is the only iron index that is able to do so. However, this index is influenced by biological factors such as gender, race, acute and chronic infections and liver disease.

Haemoglobin is the iron-containing complex in red blood cells and is the most commonly used measurement for iron status. However, this index should not be used as the only measure of iron status as haemoglobin levels for people without anaemia overlap with those of people with iron deficiency.

Serum ferritin is the best method for assessing iron deficiency. In iron-deficient individuals, serum ferritin is low in the absence of inflammation. However, inflammation can raise ferritin levels and mask iron deficiency (Kelly 2017).

2.7.5 Vitamin A Status

Assessing the vitamin A status of populations presents with many challenges. Biomarkers of vitamin A status may be classified as biological, histological, functional or biochemical tests. The wide range of biomarker tests available reflects the diverse functions of vitamin A in human physiology. The gold standard is liver biopsy, as this is the major storage organ for retinol. However, this is not a feasible method of assessing vitamin A status (Tanumihardjo 2011). Therefore, clinical signs of vitamin A deficiency were traditionally used to identify populations with a high prevalence of this problem. Initially, this was performed using the xeropthalmia classification, and now also includes assessing for night blindness and dark adaptometry. These assessments require large population studies. While these techniques may be useful for identifying clinical vitamin A deficiency, populations with a high prevalence of sub-clinical vitamin A deficiency are missed (Tanumihardjo 2004).

Alternatively, serum and breast milk retinol concentrations can be used to identify individuals and populations at risk of vitamin A deficiency. This is confounded by homeostatic control of serum retinol concentrations in healthy individuals – vitamin A deficiency does not show as low serum retinol until liver reserves are nearly depleted. Furthermore, infection lowers serum retinol and retinol binding protein concentrations, another potential confounder to assessing the true vitamin A status of individuals (Tanumihardjo 2004). To overcome these challenges, tests have been developed for identifying those with marginal vitamin A deficiency, including dose–response tests and isotope dilution assays. Apo-retinol-binding protein concentrations increase in the liver as vitamin A reserves decline, so a challenge dose of vitamin A binds to this protein, raising serum concentrations over a few hours in response and revealing low vitamin A concentrations (Tanumihardjo 2011). Stable isotopes are used as tracers to identify total body reserves and liver reserves of vitamin A. Resources available and study objectives will determine which indicator of vitamin A status is used.

2.7.6 Serum Cholesterol

Dietary fats are absorbed in the small intestine. Triglycerides are assembled and attached to very low density lipoproteins (VLDL) and chylomicrons for transport in the blood. This is because fats are hydrophobic and need to be made soluble to travel in the blood. The VLDL and chylomicrons transport fats from the digestive system to the liver. Low-density lipoproteins transport fats to the body cells where they are used for structural functions or used as an energy source for cells, or to adipose tissue for storage. High-density lipoproteins (HDL) are produced by the liver to transport fats as well. HDL collects excess cholesterol from the body cells and returns this cholesterol to the liver. VLDL, LDL and HDL are often referred to as cholesterol, and these transport proteins are measured to determine the amount of fat carried by the blood. High total cholesterol is a risk factor for cardiovascular disease. Cholesterol carriers have a high affinity for the walls of blood vessels and can build up as plaque, constricting the flow of blood within the blood vessels. Risk factors for developing this plaque include consuming a diet that is excessively high in fats, smoking, sedentary lifestyles and excessive alcohol consumption.

Cholesterol levels are monitored by measuring the concentration of total cholesterol, LDL, HDL and triglycerides in the blood. High total cholesterol is defined as a concentration greater than 5.2 mmol/dl. Low LDL cholesterol is calculated as a concentration below 3.36 mmol/dl. High HDL cholesterol is defined as a concentration greater than 1.55 mmol/dl. High triglyceride concentration is defined as a concentration above 1.69 mmol/dl.

2.7.7 Blood Glucose and HbA1c

Blood glucose rises following a meal, as carbohydrates from food are absorbed and find their way to the blood stream. When blood glucose levels rise, insulin is secreted by the pancreas, which activates receptors on cell surfaces to absorb glucose from the blood into the cells. There is then a corresponding reduction in blood glucose concentrations. Measurements of blood glucose are used to detect the presence of diabetes. Type 2 diabetes mellitus (T2DM) results from poor insulin sensitivity or low production of insulin. In T2DM, blood glucose levels remain high after a meal as the glucose is not cleared from the blood into the body cells.

Fasting blood glucose in people without diabetes ranges from 4 to 7 mmol/l and around 9 mmol/l after a meal. HbA1c is another test of blood glucose levels; however, this test is reflective of long-term blood glucose control. The typical erythrocyte has a lifespan of approximately 120 days (3 months). Glucose in the blood attaches itself to the surface of erythrocytes in a non-reversible reaction. Measuring the concentration of glucose attached to the erythrocytes gives an indication of blood glucose concentrations over a three-month period. A normal HbA1c is below 48 mmol/mol.

2.8 Clinical Assessment Indicators

Nutritional status can be assessed through clinical signs. Jeliffe and WHO (1966) defines this as a physical examination for changes related to nutritional status. These signs are typically seen in the epithelial tissue of the skin, eyes, hair and mucosa. The purpose of this form of assessment is to detect and record physical signs associated with malnutrition. Symptoms are manifestations of malnutrition which are reported by the patient. They are usually subjective, such as feelings of nausea, and are not typically observable objectively by the clinician. Clinical signs, on the other hand, are observations made by the clinician. They are more objective and immediately apparent to the observer, such as vomiting. The limitation of using clinical signs to identify malnutrition is that clinical signs and symptoms usually only appear in advanced states of malnutrition. Malnutrition may be identified earlier through anthropometric, biochemical and dietary assessments. For example, tiredness as a symptom or pallor as a sign of iron-deficiency anaemia will only manifest after a period of iron depletion when intakes do not match losses. In addition, clinical signs are often non-specific. Signs of B vitamin deficiency are often similar, such as cheilosis and angular stomatitis. Oedema may be the result of inadequate protein intakes or a symptom of wet beri–beri resulting from thiamine deficiency. The more signs of clinical deficiency a patient displays, the higher the likelihood of multiple and more severe nutritional deficiencies is. As clinical signs are non-specific, there is also a chance that physical signs observed or symptoms reported may be a result of other clinical conditions. Measles and eye conditions may present with similar changes to the relevant tissues. Environmental factors should also be considered when interpreting clinical signs and symptoms.

Clinical signs of nutritional deficiency or excess may be assessed directly by sight. These clinical signs manifest as the end result of malnutrition; therefore, malnutrition or nutrient deficiency or excess is likely to be severe before overt clinical signs are present.

Body area	Normal appearance	Signs associated with malnutrition
Hair	Shiny; firm; not easily plucked	Lack of natural shine; hair dull and dry; thin and sparse; hair fine, silky and straight; colour changes (flag sign); can easily be plucked
Face	Skin colour uni-form; smooth, pink, healthy appearance; not swollen	Skin colour loss (depigmentation); skin dark over cheeks and under eyes (malar and supra-orbital pigmentation); lump-iness or flakiness of skin of nose and mouth; swollen face; enlarged parotid glands; scaling of skin around nostrils (nasolabial seborrhoea)
Eyes	Bright, clear, shiny; no sores at corners of eyelids; mem-branes a healthy pink and are moist. No prominent blood vessels or mound of tissue or sclera	Eye membranes are pale (pale conjunc-tivae); redness of membranes (conjunc-tival injection); Bitot's spots; redness and fissuring of eyelid corners (angular palpebritis); dryness of eye membranes (conjunctival xerosis); cornea has dull appearance (corneal xerosis); comea is soft (keratomalacia); scar on cornea; ring of fine blood vessels around corner (circumcorneal injection)
Lips	Smooth, not chapped or swollen	Redness and swelling of mouth or lips (cheilosis), especially at corners of mouth (angular fissures and scars)
Tongue	Deep red in appearance; not swollen or smooth	welling; scarlet and raw tongue; magenta (purplish colour) of tongue; smooth tongue; swollen sores; hyperae-mic and hypertrophic papillae; and atrophic papillae

The strengths of clinical assessment are that they are inexpensive and yield results that are easy to interpret. However, the limitation of clinical assessment is that they may not be specific and unrelated to nutritional factors. The prevalence of clinical signs may be low except for high-risk groups. Furthermore, they may lack reliability, and there is potential for large intra-observer variability.

- **Grades of oedema**
- Depending on the presence of oedema on the different levels of the body, it is graded as follows. An increase in grades indicates an increase in the severity of oedema.
- 0 = no oedema.
- 1+ = Below the ankle (pitting pedal oedema) (mild: both feet).

- 2+ = Pitting oedema below the knee (moderate: both feet, plus lower legs, hands or lower arms).
- 3+ = Generalised oedema (severe: generalised oedema including both feet, legs, hands, arms and face).

2.8.1 Blood Pressure

Hypertension is a common public health concern. Blood pressure is read and monitored to assess the presence of hypertension. Measurements are taken of systolic and diastolic blood pressure. Systolic blood pressure is the pressure exerted by the heart on blood vessels around the body. Diastolic blood pressure is the resistance of the blood vessels against blood flow around the body. Ideally, blood pressure should be around 120/80 mmHg. Blood pressure of greater than 120/80 mmHg but lower than 140/90 mmHg is interpreted as prehypertensive, and blood pressure greater than 140/90 mmHg is hypertension. Interpreting blood pressure amongst children and adolescents is challenging as it requires the use of smoothed growth centiles for blood pressure to account for differences in height and weight at different ages. In addition, it requires multiple measurements to take an average reading.

2.9 Dietary Intake Assessment and Food Security Indicators

Food security is measured on a global scale through global food availability, on a national level by considering total food imports and local food production figures, and at household level by means of household food access and household income. The FAO method calculates food security at a national level by estimating calories available per capita using food balance sheets. Individual intake can be measured using 24-hour recall and food frequency questionnaires.

2.9.1 Dietary Assessment Methods

Food records, 24-hour recalls and food frequency questionnaires

The interviewer may influence the accuracy and quality of information collected from 24-hour recall (Castell et al. 2015). The quality of information is also affected by characteristics of the interviewee (Castell et al. 2015). Age is an important determinant of the quality of information which can be obtained. Children have challenges with independent completion of 24-hour recall, and older children complete recalls in a shorter time than younger children (Raffoul et al. 2019). Thirteen year olds took an average 31 minutes to complete a self-administered digital 24-hour recall compared with 52 minutes for ten year olds (Raffoul et al. 2019). Children tend to overestimate the total calories eaten but underestimate intake of foods such as cookies and juice (Raffoul et al. 2019). Children have limited food recognition skills, memory constraints, an undeveloped concept of time and short concentration spans that affect their ability to undertake 24-hour recalls (Foster and Bradley 2018).

Interview support tools affect the quality of information obtained (Castell et al. 2015). Kirkpatrick et al. (2016) have demonstrated that using digital images improved the accuracy of 24-hour recall. The images were tailored to different types and forms of food, which raised the quality of the estimations of oral intake (Kirkpatrick et al. 2016). Digital or computer-based tools for self-administering 24-hour recalls may help to reduce interviewer bias (Castell et al. 2015). However, these methods also have the disadvantage of costs for equipment and programs, and may be difficult to administer in populations who are unfamiliar with technology or who require assistance such as the elderly (Castell et al. 2015).

The use of 24-hour recall has advantages over other dietary assessment methods. Users report that is a faster method than food frequency questionnaires. According to interviewees, 24-hour recall gives a better indication of typical dietary patterns than food frequency questionnaires (DeBiasse et al. 2017). However, 24-hour recall has limitations. The method relies on the short-term memory abilities of interviewees, which may be problematic in the very young or elderly. It also depends on the interviewer's ability to describe ingredients, food preparation techniques and dish or portion sizes. The technique requires trained interviewers. A once-off 24 hour recall will not indicate usual dietary intake (Castell et al. 2015). Food records and 24-hour recall both underestimate energy intake by approximately 30% when compared with doubly labelled water estimation of energy consumption (Lopes et al. 2016).

The coding system and computer software allow for statistical analysis (Castell et al. 2015).

Food and beverage composition tables affect quality (Castell et al. 2015).

2.9.2 Assessing the Nutritional Status of Populations

The nutritional status of populations is assessed by nutritional surveys and surveillance. Assessing the nutritional status of populations has clinical, public health and research applications (Patterson and Pietinen 2004). Policy makers, programme managers, researchers and advocates involved in the nutrition field require accurate data on nutritional status (WHO and UNICEF 2009). The assessment of populations estimates the mean measures of nutritional status for patient groups. This allows clinicians to characterise the nutritional status of patient populations (Patterson and Pietinen 2004). Nutritional surveillance is a public health method of monitoring nutritional status over time. Nutritional surveillance allows policy makers to identify nutritional inadequacies in a population, assess the impact of public health interventions and act as an early warning system for crises (Mason et al. 1984).

Anthropometric indicators of nutritional status are routinely collected for nutritional surveys to assess the health of populations. Weight, height and waist circumference are the basic anthropometric indicators recommended for nutritional surveillance of non-communicable diseases by the World Health Organization (2005). The World Health Organisation and UNICEF (2019) recommend measuring weight, height or length and age amongst children younger than five years old for nutrition surveillance.

By measuring weight and height, researchers and policy makers are able to assess BMI for populations. High BMI and prevalence estimates for overweight and obesity can give an indication of the risk of complications such as hypertension, heart disease and diabetes for the population. This is valuable information when developing national health budgets and deciding on the allocation of resources. The addition of waist circumference increases the accuracy of the estimations, as measures of central obesity are better indicators of cardiovascular disease risk. Waist and height taken together may be used to calculate WHR, as described above, which further improves the accuracy of measures of heart disease risk. The addition of hip circumference allows researchers to assess the mean waist-to-hip ratio. MUAC has not been included as an indicator for the Sustainable Development Goals.

24-hour recall is used in nutritional surveillance programmes in the United States of America, Australia and the United Kingdom. The STEPS tool (World Health Organization 2005) advises monitoring fruit and vegetable consumption as a core behavioural indicator, and oil and fat use as an expanded item. The limitations of this technique have already been described, along with some potential strategies for their improvement. Many of these interviews are carried out over the telephone for the purpose of conducting nutrition surveillance. This means that the accuracy of the assessment relies even more heavily on the interviewer. There is less opportunity for using tools such as digital images in this setting.

Food security is monitored using the food insecurity experience scale (FIES) (FAO 2018).

2.9.3 Assessing the Nutritional Status of Individuals

The nutritional status of individuals is evaluated through screening and by nutritional assessment. Nutritional screening and assessment are often thought of as interchangeable terms; however, screening and assessment are two different processes (Correia 2018). Nutritional screening gives an indication of risk for a nutritional condition, while assessment provides a nutritional diagnosis (Correia 2018). Nutritional screening compares observed measurements with predetermined cut-off values that correspond to malnutrition risk (Gibson 2005).

2.10 An Introduction to WHO Anthro – Online Anthropometric Software

WHO Anthro is a free, open access program that can be downloaded from the WHO website. It allows health workers to calculate the Z-scores of anthropometric measurements of children and analyse individuals and trends for large samples. This section includes a worked example and resources.

WHO Anthro is software that was developed to facilitate the application of the WHO child growth standards in individuals and populations of children up to the age of five years (WHO 2007). A nutritional survey module forms part of the specific functions of the programme (WHO 2007). Calculating the Z-score for each individual participant in a survey would be extremely time consuming. The great advantage of the WHO Anthro software is that it allows researchers and health workers to convert weight and height into Z-scores for analysis. Researchers and health workers may be interested in this information in order to evaluate prevalence rates for underweight, stunting, wasting or overweight, or use the data to assess correlations between childhood anthropometry.

The software developed by the World Health Organisation for analysing anthropometric data for children younger than five years is available from https://www.who.int/childgrowth/software/en. WHO Anthro makes use of shinyapps for R. R is a free statistical analysis software package that requires researchers to have an understanding of coding to perform statistical analyses. Shinyapps are applications that make use of R but are more user friendly.

The software is available to use online or offline. In the online version, the user uploads data in a .csv file, which is then analysed, and the results can be downloaded. In the offline version, the user downloads software that can be used as an application.

Open the file and you will see that data has been collected on children's weight and height measurements, age and gender. The online software will map the data according to variables required to calculate Z-scores, including age, sex, weight and height. Age can be calculated from the child's date of birth and date of visit by the data collector. In our version of the data capture spreadsheet, we need to ensure that the file is compatible with the data mapping software. Select the column

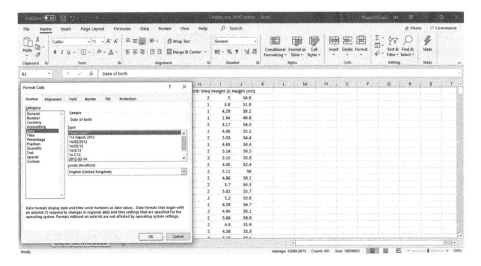

Figure 2.8: Formatting the date for WHO Anthro.

Source: World Health Organization (WHO).

'Date of birth', right click on the column, and select 'format cells'. Under date, select the option for the date format 'dd/mm/yyyy'. Follow the same procedure for the Date of visit column, as shown in Figure 2.8.

To convert the file into a form that is accessible to WHO Anthro, select File, Save as and then choose the type of file you would like to save the document as by clicking on the drop-down arrow beneath the file name. Select .csv (comma delineated file). The online software will not recognise the file if there are any spaces in the file name, so replace the spaces with underscores ('_') and change the '2' in the title to 'two'. Now save the file. This is the version that will be uploaded to the online software. To use the online version, follow the link above and select 'online version'. Scroll to the bottom of the page and select 'Go to the Antho Survey Analyser'. A new page will appear, with an area for uploading your .csv file. You can upload your data by selecting browse and locating the file to upload, or by dragging the file from its folder to the upload area.

Now that the file is uploaded, we need to map the variables so that Antho knows what to use to calculate the Z-scores for the data.

On the left-hand side of the page, select the data of birth drop-down arrow under 'Age mapping' and select 'date.of.birth' as shown in Figure 2.9. Note that the spaces in the column name have been replaced with full stops. Choose 'date.of.visit' for the date of visit variable. Choose 'Gender' for the sex variable, 'Weight..kg.' for the weight variable and 'Height..cm.' for the length or height variable. The analysis has already been taking place as we mapped our variables.

Go to the top of the page and select the Z-scores tab. Here you will see that a Z-score has been calculated for each participant. The Z-scores can

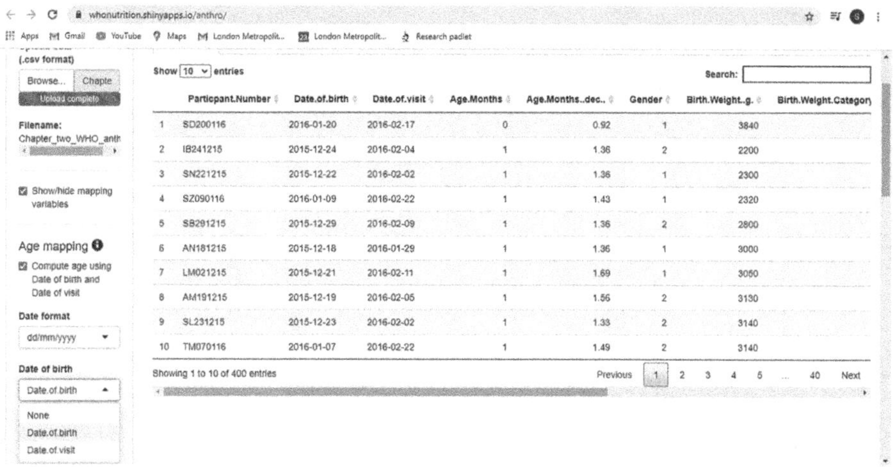

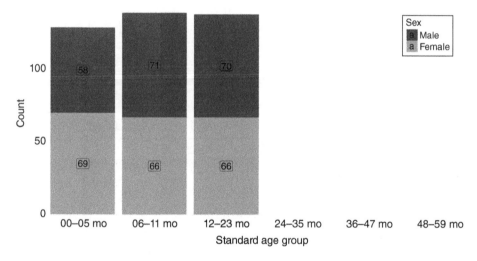

Figure 2.9: Selecting columns as variables on WHO Anthro.
Source: WORLD HEALTH ORGANIZATION (WHO)

Figure 2.10: Descriptive data outputs from WHO Anthro.

be downloaded for further analysis using programs such as Microsoft Excel, SPSS and Stata. The column in the downloaded file named 'zlen' presents the length-for-age Z-score for each participant, 'zwei' is the weight-for-age Z-score and 'zwfl' is the weight-for-length Z-score.

The data quality analysis tab provides information on the distributions of the data, missing data, Z-score distribution and summary data. This information can be viewed by selecting the tabs under the data quality analysis tab. Specific variables can be chosen to view the distributions of data such as gender, age group, weight and length-summary data, which is commonly reported in the descriptive statistics in scientific reports on anthropometric data (Figure 2.10).

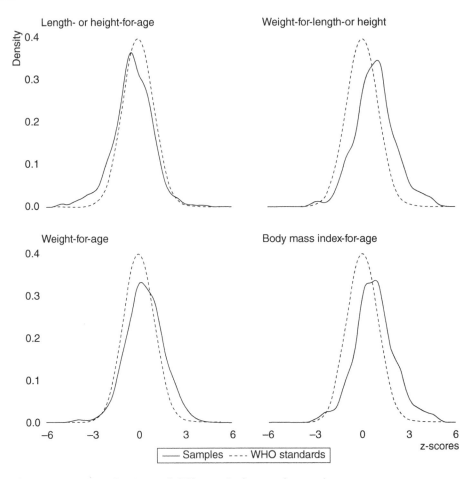

Figure 2.11: Distributions of different indexes of growth.

The *Z*-score distribution of the data can also be viewed (Figure 2.11). This visual representation can be used to look for patterns and trends in the data. The data can also be stratified using variables such as age and sex to gain further insights.

Annex: Summary of Recommended Data Quality Checks

The Working Group (WG) on Anthropometry Data Quality recommendation is that data quality be assessed and reported based on assessment on the following seven parameters: (i) completeness, (ii) sex ratio, (iii) age distribution, (iv) digit preference of heights and weights, (v) implausible *Z*-score values, (vi) standard deviation of *Z*-scores and (vii) normality of *Z*-scores.

The WG recommends that (i) data quality checks should not be considered in isolation, (ii) formal tests or scoring should not be conducted and (iii) the checks should be used to help users identify issues with the data quality to improve interpretation of the malnutrition estimates from the survey. Although not exhaustive, a summary of details on the various checks is provided below to help their use. Full details and more comprehensive guidance, including on how to calculate, can be found at the full report on the WG's recommendations.[1]

i. **Completeness: Although not all statistics are included in the WHO Anthro Survey Analyser, report on structural integrity of the aspects listed below should be included in the final report:**
   - PSUs: % of selected PSUs that were visited.
   - Households: % of selected households in the PSUs interviewed or recorded as not interviewed (specifying why).
   - Household members: % of household rosters that were completed.
   - Children: % of all eligible children are interviewed and measured, or recorded as not interviewed or measured (specifying why), with no duplicate cases.
   - Dates of birth: % of dates of birth for all eligible children that were complete.

ii. **Sex ratio:**
   - What – Ratio of girls to boys in the survey and compare to expected for country. The observed ratios should be compared to the expected patterns based on reliable sources.
   - Why – To identify potential selection biases.

iii. **Age distribution:**
   - What – Age distributions by age in completed years (6 bars weighted), months (72 bars) and calendar month of birth (12 bars), as histograms.
   - Why – To identify potential selection biases or misreporting.

iv. **Height and weight digit preference:**
   - What – Terminal digits as well as whole number integer distributions through histograms.
   - Why – Digit preference may be a tell-tale sign of data fabrication or inadequate care and attention during data collection and recording. When possible, it should be presented by team or other relevant disaggregation categories.

[1] Working Group on Anthropometric Data Quality, for the WHO–UNICEF Technical Expert Advisory Group on Nutrition Monitoring (TEAM). Recommendations for improving the quality of anthropometric data and its analysis and reporting. Available at http://www.who.int/nutrition/team (under 'Technical reports and papers').

v. **Implausible *Z*-score values:**
  - What – The % of cases outside of WHO flags[2] for each HAZ, WHZ and WAZ.
  - Why – A percent above 1% can be indicative of potential data quality issues in measurements or age determination. It should be presented by team or other relevant disaggregation categories.

vi. **Standard deviations:**
  - What – SD for each HAZ, WHZ and WAZ.
  - Why – Large SDs may be a sign of data quality problems and/or population heterogeneity. It is unclear what causes SD's size, and more research is needed to determine appropriate interpretation. It should be noted that SDs are typically wider for HAZ than WHZ or WAZ, and that HAZ SD is typically widest in youngest (0–5 months) and increases as children age through to five years. No substantial difference should be observed between boys and girls. It should be presented by team or other relevant disaggregation categories.

vii. **Checks of normality:**
  - What – Measures of asymmetry (skew) and tailedness (kurtosis) of HAZ, WHZ and WAZ, as well as density plots.
  - Why – General assumption that three indices are normally distributed but unclear if applicable to populations with varying patterns of malnutrition. One can use the rule of thumb ranges of <-0.5 or $>+0.5$ for skewness to indicate asymmetry and <2 or >4 for kurtosis to indicate heavy or light tails. Further research needed to understand patterns in different contexts. Anyhow the comparisons amongst the distribution by disaggregation categories might help with the interpretation of results.

References

Ali, E., Zachariah, R., Shams, Z. et al. (2013). Is mid-upper arm circumference alone sufficient for deciding admission to a nutritional programme for childhood severe acute malnutrition in Bangladesh? *Trans. R. Soc. Trop. Med. Hyg.* 107: 319–323.

Alvarez-Uria G, Midde M, Pakam R, Bachu L, Naik PK (2012). Effect of formula feeding and breast feeding on child growth, infant mortality, and HIV transmission in children born to HIV-infected pregnant women who receive triple antiretroviral therapy in a resource-limited setting: Data from an HIV cohort study in India. ISRN Paediatrics.

---

[2] WHO Anthro Software for personal computers – Manual (2011). Available at http://www.who.int/childgrowth/software/anthro_pc_manual_v322.pdf?ua=1.

Ashwell, M. and Gibson, S. (2016). Waist-to-height ratio as an indicator of 'early health risk': simpler and more predictive than using a 'matrix' based on BMI and waist circumference. *BMJ Open* 6: e010159.

Blanck, H.M., Bowman, B.A., Cooper, G.R. et al. (2003). Laboratory issues: Use of nutritional biomarkers. *J. Nutr.* 133 (3): 888S–894S.

Briend, A. and Prinzo, Z.W. (2009). Dietary management of moderate malnutrition: Time for change. *Food Nutr. Bull.* 30 (3): S265–S266.

Briend, A. and Zimicki, S. (1986). Validation of arm circumferene as an indicator of risk of death in one to four year old children. *Nutr. Res.* 6 (3): 249–261.

Briend, A., Maire, B., Fontaine, O., and Garenne, M. (2015). Mid-upper arm circumference and weight-for-height to identify high-risk malnourished under-five children. *Matern. Child Nutr.* 8 (1): 130–133.

Burden, S.T., Bodey, S., Bradburn, Y.J. et al. (2001). Validation of a nutrition screening tool: Testing the reliability and validity. *J. Hum. Nutr. Diet.* 14 (4): 269–275.

Castell, G.S., Serra-Majem, L., and Ribas-Barba, L. (2015). What and how much do we eat? 24 hour dietary recall method. *Nutr. Hosp.* 31 (S3): 46–48.

Centre for Disease Control (2007). National Health and Nutrition Examination Survey Anthropometry Procedures Manual, 2007.

Cloete, I., Daniels, L., Jordaan, J. et al. (2013). Knowledge and perceptions of nursing staff on the new road to health booklet growth charts in primary healthcare clinics in the Tygerberg subdistrict of the Cape Town metropole district. *S. Afr. J. Clin. Nutr.* 26 (3).

Cole, T.J. and Lobstein, T. (2012). Extended international (IOTF) body mass index cut-offs for thinness, overweight and obesity. *Paediatr. Obesity* 7 (4): 284–294.

Correia, M.I.T.D. (2018). Nutrition screening vs nutrition assessment: what is the difference? *Nutr. Clin. Pract.* 33 (1): 62–72.

Courtinhop, T., Goel, K., de Sa, D. et al. (2011). Central obesity and survival in subjects with coronary artery disease: a systematic review of the literature and collaborative analysis with individual subject data. *J. Am. Coll. Cardiol.* 57 (19): 1877–1886.

Dairo, M.D., Fatokun, M.E., and Kuti, M. (2012). Reliability of the mid upper arm circumference for the assessment of wasting among children aged 12-59 months in urban Ibadan, Nigeria. *Int. J. Biomed. Sci.* 8 (2): 140–143.

De Onis, M. (2015). The WHO child growth standards. *World Rev. Nutr. Diet.* 113: 278–294.

De Onis, M., Yip, R., and Mei, Z. (1997). The development of MUAC-for-age reference data recommended by a WHO Expert Committee. *Bull. World Health Organ.* 75 (1): 11–18.

De Onis, M., Garza, C., Victora, C.G. et al. (2004a). The WHO Multicentre Growth Reference Study (MGRS): rationale, planning and implementation. *Food Nutr. Bull.* 25 (1): S21–S26.

De Onis, M., Winjhoven, T.M.A., and Onyango, A.W. (2004b). Worldwide practice in child growth monitoring. *J. Paediatr. Dent.* 144 (4): 461–465.

De Onis, M., Onyango, A., Borghi, E., Siyam, A., Nishida, C., Nishida, J. (2006). *WHO Child Growth Standards: Length/Height-for-Age, Weight-for-Age, Weight-for-Length, Weight-for Height and Body Mass Index-for-Age: Methods and Development.* Geneva: World Health Organisation.

De Onis, M., Garza, C., Onyango, A.W., and Borghi, E. (2007). Comparison of the WHO child growth standards and the CDC 2000 growth charts. *J. Nutr.* 137 (1): 144–148.

De Onis, M., Onyango, A., Borghi, E. et al. (2012). *Worldwide Implementation of the WHO Child Growth Standards*. Public Health Nutrition.

DeBiasse, M.A., Bowen, D.J., Quatromoni, P.A. et al. (2017). Feasibility and acceptability of dietary intake assessment via 24-hour recall and food frequency questionnaire among women with low socioeconomic status. *J. Acad. Nutr. Diet.* 118 (2): 301–307.

Dibley, M.J., Goldsby, J.B., Staehling, N.W., and Trowbridge, F.L. (1987). Development of normalized curves for the international growth reference: historical and technical considerations. *Am. J. Clin. Nutr.* 46: 736–748.

Duggan, M.B. (2013). Anthropometry as a tool for measuring malnutrition: impact of the new WHO growth standards and reference. *Ann. Trop. Paediatr.* 30 (1): 1–17.

FAO (2018). Voices of the hungry: The Food Insecurity Experience Scale. Available from: https://www.fao.org/in-action/voices-of-the-hungry/fies/en/

Foster, E. and Bradley, J. (2018). Methodological considerations and future insights for 24-hour dietary recall assessment in children. *Nutr. Res.* 5: 1–11.

Ganz, T. (2003). Hepcidin, a key regulator of iron metabolism and mediator of anemia of inflammation. *Blood* 102 (3): 783–788.

Garrow, J.S. (1988). *Obesity and Related Diseases*, 1–16. London: Churchill Livingstone.

Gibson, R.E. (2005). *Principles of Nutrition Assessment*, 2e. Oxford: Oxford University Press.

Hall, A., Oirere, M., Thurstans, S. et al. (2011). The practical challenges of evaluating a blanket emergency feeding programme in Northern Kenya. *PLoS One* 6 (10): e26854.

Huxley, R., Mendis, S., Zheleznyakov, E. et al. (2010). Body mass index, waist circumference and waist:hip ratio – a review of the literature. *Eur. J. Clin. Nutr.* 64 (1): 16–22.

Janssen, I., Katzmarzyk, P.T., and Ross, R. (2004). Waist circumference and not body mass index explains obesity-related health risk. *Am. J. Clin. Nutr.* 79 (3): 379–384.

Jeliffe, D.B. and World Health Organisation (1966). The assessment of the nutritional status of the community (with special reference to field surveys in developing regions of the world. *World Health Organ.* https://apps.who.int/iris/handle/10665/41780

Joseph, B., Rebello, A., Kullu, P., and Raj, V.D. (2002). Prevalence of malnutrition in Karnataka, South India: a comparison of anthropometric indicators. *J. Health Popul. Nutr.* 20 (3): 239–244.

Kelly, A.U. (2017). Interpreting iron studies. *Br. Med. J.* 357: 2513.

Kirkpatrick, S.I., Potischman, N., Dodd, K.W. et al. (2016). The use of digital images in 24-hour recall may lead to less misestimation of portion size compared with traditional interviewer-administered recalls. *J. Nutr.* 146 (12): 2567–2573.

Laillou, A., Prak, S., de Groot, R. et al. (2014). Optimal Screening of Children with Acute Malnutrition Requires a Change in Current WHO Guidelines as MUAC and WHZ Identify Different Patient Groups. *PLoS One* (9, 7): e101159. pmid:24983995.

Lean, M.E.J., Han, T.S., and Morrison, C.E. (1995). Waist circumference as a measure for identifying need for weight management. *Br. Med. J.* 311: 158.

Lopes, T.S., Luiz, R.R., Hoffman, D.J. et al. (2016). Misreport of energy intake assessed with food records and 24-hour recalls compared with total energy expenditures estimated with DLW. *Eur. J. Clin. Nutr.* 70: 259–1264.

Martorell, R. and Young, M.F. (2012). Patterns of stunting and wasting: potential explanatory factors. *Adv. Nutr.* 3: 227–233.

Mason, J.B., Habicht, J.P., Tabatabai, H., and Valverde, V. (1984). *Nutritional Surveillance.* Geneva: World Health Organisation.

McCarthy, H.D. (2014). Measuring growth and obesity across childhood and adolescence. *Proc. Nutr. Soc.* 73 (2): 210–217.

Ononamadu, C.J., Ezekwisili, C.N., Onyenkwu, O.F. et al. (2017). Comparative analysis of anthropometric indices of obesity as correlates and potential predictors of risk for hypertension and prehypertension in a population in Nigeria. *Cardiovasc. J. Afr.* 28 (2): 92–99.

Patterson, R.E. and Pietinen, P. (2004). *Assessment of Nutritional Status in Individuals and Populations. Public Health Nutrition.* Oxford: Blackwell Science.

Raffoul, A., Hobin, E.P., Sacco, J.E. et al. (2019). School-age children can recall some foods and beverages consumed the prior day using the self-administered 24-hour dietary assessment tool (ASA24) without assistance. *J. Nutr.* 149 (6): 1019–1026.

Retamal, R. and Nicholas Mascie-Taylor, C.G. (2019). Trends of weight gain and prevalence of overweight and obesity from birth to three years of age. *Obesity Res. Clin. Res.* 13: 6–11.

Romero-Corral, A., Montori, V.M., Somers, V.K. et al. (2006). Association of body weight with total mortality and with cardiovascular events in coronary artery disease: a systematic review of cohort studies. *Lancet* 368: 666–678.

Semba, R.D. and Bloem, M.W. (2008). *Nutrition and Health in Developing Countries,* 2e. New Jersey: Humana Press.

Tanumihardjo, S.A. (2004). Assessing vitamin A status: past, present and future. *J. Nutr.* 134 (1): 290S–293S.

Tanumihardjo, S.A. (2011). Vitamin A: biomarkers of nutrition for development. *Am. J. Clin. Nutr.* 94 (2): 658S–665S.

Thomas, P.C., Marino, L.K., Williams, S.A., and Beattie, R.M. (2016). Outcome of nutritional screening in the acute setting. *Arch. Dis. Child.* 101: 1119–1124.

Vasundhara, D., Hemalatha, R., Sharma, S. et al. (2020). Maternal MUAC and fetal outcome in an Indian tertiary care hospital: a prospective observational study. *Matern. Child Nutr.* 16 (2): e12902.

WHO (2006). *WHO Multicentre Growth Reference Study Group: WHO Child Growth Standards: Length/Height for Age, Weight for Age, Weight for Length, Weight for Height and Body Mass Index for Age: Methods and Development.* Geneva: World Health Organisation.

WHO and UNICEF (2009). *WHO Growth Standards and the Identification of Severe Acute Malnutrition in Infants and Children: A Joint Statement by the World Health Organisation and United Nations Children's Fund.* Geneva, Switzerland: World Health Organisation.

WHO Anthro for mobile devices version 2 (2007). *Software for Assessing Growth and Development of the World's Children.* Geneva: WHO.

WHO (2013). Guideline: *Updates on the management of severe acute malnutrition in infants and children.* Geneva: World Health Organization.

World Health Organisation (2008). *Waist Circumference and Wasit-Hip Ratio: Report of a WHO Expert Consultation, Geneva, 8–11 December 2008.* Geneva: World Health Organisation.

World Health Organisation and UNICEF (2019). *Recommendations for Data Collection, Analysis and Reporting on Anthropometric Indicators in Children under 5 Years Old.* Geneva: World Health Organisation and United Nations Childrens Fund (UNICEF).

World Health Organization (2005). *Noncommunicable Diseases and Mental Health Cluster (2005) WHO STEPS Surveillance Manual: The WHO STEPwise Approach to Chronic Disease Risk Factor Surveillance.* Geneva: World Health Organization.

3 Nutrition Surveillance

3.1 Introduction

Public health surveillance is used to track health indicators. Nutritionists and other public health professionals often use nutrition surveillance reports to identify trends in diet-related health, plan their interventions and evaluate their success.

The number of empirical studies on priority setting in developing countries is increasing (Youngkong et al. 2009). Public Health England states the importance of public health surveillance in their statement 'surveillance is a core function for Public Health England and ensures that we have the right information available to use at the right time to inform public health decisions and actions'.

'Public health surveillance is the continuous, systematic collection, analysis and interpretation of health-related data needed for the planning, implementation and evaluation of public health practice. Such surveillance can: serve as an early warning system for impending public health emergencies; document the impact of an intervention, or track progress towards specified goals; and monitor and clarify the epidemiology of health problems, to allow priorities to be set and to inform public health policy and strategies' (WHO definition).

3.2 The Uses of Nutritional Survey Data

Nutritional survey data is used for three main purposes: to serve as an early warning system, to inform policy and programmes and to evaluate programmes and interventions.

Nutritional surveillance is used for long-term monitoring of public health (Mason et al. 1984). Nutrition surveillance provides an ongoing description of nutrition-related conditions in a population. It may describe specific sub-groups. It is used for planning, analysing the effects of policies

Nutrition and Global Health, First Edition. Shawn W. McLaren.
© 2023 John Wiley & Sons Ltd. Published 2023 by John Wiley & Sons Ltd.

and for predicting future trends (Mason et al. 1984). Nutrition surveillance is used for evaluating programme impact through monitoring changes in nutrition indicators after initiating nutrition programmes (Mason et al. 1984). In an example from South Africa, a study has showed a high rate of vitamin A deficiency (which identified vitamin A deficiency as a problem). Interventions were planned, and vitamin A supplementation was initiated in 2002 and food fortification with vitamin A in 2003 (Republic of South Africa 2003). The National Food Consumption Survey (NCFS) (Labadarios et al. 2005) reported that vitamin A deficiency was prevalent among 63.6% of the under-five population in 2005. By 2013 (Shisana et al. 2013), the prevalence reported by nutrition surveillance had improved to 43.6%. By allowing the monitoring of trends, nutrition surveillance can act as a timely warning and intervention system. This can contribute to the prevention of epidemic inadequacies in food consumption (Mason et al. 1984).

3.3 Competing National Health Priorities and Their Effect on the Focus of Nutritional Survey Data

Nutritional surveillance potentially includes all parts of the food system – a cumbersome task. How do countries and aid organisations select the indicators that will best inform their decisions? Criteria include cost-effectiveness, severity of the problem and the size of potential benefits. The scope and scale of a nutrition surveillance programme is influenced by resources available as well as factors such as geographic size of the country, strength of coverage and their methods for data collection.

Nutrition surveillance potentially concerns all steps of the food system (Mason et al. 1984) (Figure 3.1). The food system includes food production and agriculture, processing, distribution and food consumption (Tansey and Worsley 1995). The food system is vast and every living individual is involved. The degree of involvement varies depending on the individual, with more direct involvement from famers, caterers and distributors. However, consumers and the end use of products play a crucial important role in the buyer–driver commodity food system (Fold 2002; Tansey and Worsley 1995). Youngkong et al. (2009) identified that involving different stakeholders as respondents was an important methical technique commonly employed in empirical policy-setting studies in developing countries. The food system is also a dynamic system and responds to the changing demand, resources and structure of society. Economic factors such as urbanisation, advances in agricultural and food science, environmental impact and food policy affect the food system (Tansey and

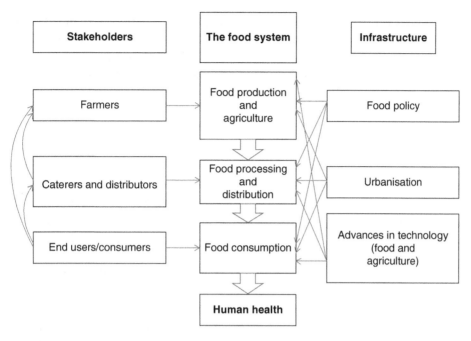

Figure 3.1: The complexity of the food system.

Worsley 1995), and ultimately have an impact on human health (Anand et al. 2015).

The result is that nutrition surveillance involves collecting a large amount of data from a wide range of industries and consumers (Mason et al. 1984). Therefore, public health planners are required to prioritise the types of information that will be most useful to them. Only data that is needed to make decisions on public policies and programmes to ensure adequate nutrition of the population is included in a nutritional survey (Mason et al. 1984).

Deciding where to allocate resources is necessary in all health care systems. Cost-effectiveness, the size of individual benefits and severity of disease have been identified as important criteria in decision making (Defechereux et al. 2012).

Nutritional surveillance surveys include indicators of micronutrient status of children, pregnant women, infant and child feeding practices, anthropometry of children 0–59 months, underweight, stunting and wasting. These indicators are generally universal (Friedman 2014).

Countries in low- and middle-income countries (LMIC) such as Ethiopia and Somalia prioritise indicators of child health, including mortality 0–59 months, causes of mortality 0–59 months, morbidity 0–59 months, measles and BCG vaccine coverage and vitamin A coverage in the last 6 months in their nutritional surveillance systems (Friedman 2014). More developed countries such as Kuwait and Palestinian territories include additional indicators more aligned with the health of adults and the elderly, including anaemia, blood glucose of diabetics, cholesterol in adults, obesity rates, physical activity rates and TV and computer habits (Friedman 2014). These differences may be attributed to factors such as the geographical size of the survey area, strength of coverage and method of data collection.

3.4 Methods of Nutritional Surveillance

Surveys may use qualitative or quantitative methods, or a combination of the two. Primary data is collected from repeated cross-sectional surveys, while secondary data can come from monitoring health facility statistics, feeding centres and mass screening programmes. There are advantages and disadvantages of both methods.

Studies use both qualitative and quantitative techniques, or a combination of these (Youngkong et al. 2009).

Primary data is collected using repeated cross-sectional surveys, community-based sentinel monitoring and collection of data from schools. Secondary data comes from feeding centres' health facilities and community-based data collection including mass screenings for malnutrition in children (Tuffrey and Hall 2016).

The WHO has produced a nutrition surveillance tool to assist countries in prioritising risk factors for nutritional problems for monitoring. This tool named 'STEPS' divides monitoring into three categories, namely behavioural, physical and biochemical measurements. Behavioural items include basic demographic information such as age, sex, literacy and highest level of education, as well as tobacco use, alcohol consumption, fruit and vegetable consumption and physical activity. These factors can be expanded to include more detailed demographic information about years spent in education, ethnicity, marital status, employment status, smokeless tobacco use, drinking over the past seven days, history of blood pressure treatment for raised blood pressure and history of diabetes or treatment for diabetes. Optional modules include monitoring mental health, intentional or unintentional injury and violence and oral health. It may also include an objective measure of physical activity behaviour. Core physical measurements recommended for nutritional surveillance include weight and height, waist circumference and blood pressure. This may be expanded to include hip circumference and heart rate (Weight and height as measures are used to calculate body mass index, waist circumference is a measure of central obesity - slightly more indicative of non-communicable disease risk and waist-to-hip ratio as an even more detailed indicator). Optional modules for physical measurements include skinfold thickness and assessment of physical fitness. Core biochemical measurements include fasting blood sugar and total cholesterol, which may be expanded to include fasting high-density lipoprotein (HDL) cholesterol. Optional modules include an oral glucose tolerance test, urine examination and salivary cotinine.

The frequency of data collection for nutrition surveillance varies greatly depending on the nutrition surveillance system. Nutritional surveillance data may be collected continuously or at planned intervals. Community-based sentinel sites collect data continuously, while repeated nutrition surveys collect data at intervals. Continuous data may also be repeated from health clinics or from feeding programme admissions. Data may be collected from mass screenings. The frequency of data collection may be determined by the purpose of the nutritional survey as described previously – continuous data might be used to monitor and clarify the epidemiology of health problems or serve as an early warning system for impending public health emergencies. Data collected at intervals allows priorities to be set and to inform public health policy and strategies, in part due to the more reliable nature of the data collected. The frequency of data collection may also be influenced by the resources available to policy makers.

Repeated sample surveys require staff with expertise in survey design and data analysis. The technical designs of repeated sample surveys are generally strong. The data collected is representative on a national scale and offers an opportunity for analysis at a subnational level as well. Technical assistance in survey design and data analysis is available from international organisations, including the WHO, UNICEF and CDC. External expertise is often critical to the success of repeated sample surveys. Surveys of this type are sometimes difficult to carry out, especially in countries with poor infrastructure, geographically dispersed populations and in regions with pockets of insecurity. These surveys generally cost more than other data collection methods.

Data collected from public health clinics or sentinel sites are easier to collect and analyse. Sampling is simplified, as patients present themselves to the sites; however, this means that the results are associated with the limitations of convenience samples. These include limited generalisability of the findings of this form of surveillance. As an example, patterns in childhood malnutrition might represent patterns among children who attend or have access to primary healthcare facilities, but are not representative of children who do not have access.

Geographic coverage is another important aspect of nutritional surveillance. Surveyors may attempt to collect data in all subnational regions in order to build nationally and regionally representative samples. Policy makers and health planners may choose to target areas that are highly vulnerable to food insecurity only.

There is large variation in sample size for nutritional surveys between countries. The sample size is generally presented as the number of individuals included or as the number of households included in the survey. The sample size may range from several hundred households as in the case of Nicaragua ($n = 540$) to thousands of households as collected in the Democratic Republic of Congo ($n = 1250$) or Uganda ($n = 3420$). Data is generally collected on infants and children from birth to 59 months in all countries.

3.5 Analysing Health Data

Public health data is used by health workers, researchers and epidemiologists to track changes in key health indicators. Programmes including Microsoft Excel and IBM's SPSS can be used to make sense of public health data. This section provides worked examples with resources.

Scenario 1:
National surveys including those carried out by the Demographic and Health Survey (DHS) often include information about child feeding practices. Data on child feeding practices can be used to track progress towards key indicators, which in turn can inform policy makers and health workers. In the first worked example, we use fictitious raw data to monitor progress towards key indicators of infant and young child feeding. The indicators are as follows:

1. Early initiation of breastfeeding
2. Exclusive breastfeeding under six months
3. Exclusive breastfeeding (infants 4–5 months)
4. Continued breastfeeding at one year
5. Introduction of solid, semi-solid or soft foods
6. Minimum dietary diversity
7. Minimum meal frequency
8. Minimum acceptable diet

More information on infant and young child feeding can be found in the chapter on Maternal and Child Nutrition. The data presented here is intended to represent interval survey data, or primary data.

Indicator 1: Early initiation of breastfeeding
Proportion of children born in the last 24 months who were put to the breast within one hour of birth.

Children born in the last 24 months who were put to the breast within one hour of birth/children born in the last 24 months.

Indicator 2: Exclusive breastfeeding under six months
Proportion of infants 0–5 months of age who are fed exclusively with breast milk.

Infants 0–5 months of age who received only breast milk during the previous day/infants 0–5 months of age.

Indicator 3: Exclusive breastfeeding (infants 4–5 months)
Proportion of infants 4–5 months of age who are fed exclusively with breast milk.

Infants 4–5 months of age who received only breast milk during the previous day/infants 4–5 months of age.

Indicator 4: Continued breastfeeding at one year
Proportion of children 12–15 months of age who are fed breast milk.

Children 12–15 months of age who received breast milk during the previous day/children 12–15 months of age.

Indicator 5: Introduction of solid, semi-solid or soft foods
Proportion of infants 6–8 months of age who receive solid, semi-solid or soft foods.

Infants 6–8 months of age who received solid, semi-solid or soft foods during the previous day/infants 6–8 months of age.

Indicator 6: Minimum dietary diversity
Proportion of children 6–23 months of age who receive foods from four or more food groups.

Children 6–23 months of age who received foods from ≥4 food groups during the previous day/children 6–23 months of age.

The sample universe for this indicator is last born children 6–23 months of age living with their mothers.
- The seven food groups used for calculation of this indicator are as follows:
  - Grains, roots and tubers
  - Legumes and nuts
  - Dairy products (milk, yogurt and cheese)
  - Flesh foods (meat, fish, poultry and liver/organ meats)
  - Eggs
  - Vitamin A rich fruits and vegetables
  - Other fruits and vegetables

Indicator 7: Minimum meal frequency

Proportion of breastfed and non-breastfed children 6–23 months of age, who receive solid, semi-solid or soft foods (but also including milk feeds for non-breastfed children) the minimum number of times or more.

This indicator is calculated from the following two fractions:

Breastfed children 6–23 months of age who received solid, semi-solid or soft foods the minimum number of times or more during the previous day/breastfed children 6–23 months of age.

Non-breastfed children 6–23 months of age who received solid, semi-solid or soft foods or milk feeds the minimum number of times or more during the previous day/non-breastfed children 6–23 months of age.

The sample universe for this indicator is last-born children 6–23 months of age living with their mothers.

- For breastfed children, the minimum meal frequency is defined as two times for infants 6–8 months and three times for children 9–23 months.
- For non-breastfed children, the minimum meal frequency is defined as four times for children 6–23 months.
- Values for this indicator could not be calculated for non-breastfed children because the DHS questionnaires did not include a question about the frequency of milk feeds.

Indicator 8: Minimum acceptable diet

Proportion of children 6–23 months of age who receive a minimum acceptable diet (apart from breast milk). The indicator is calculated from the following two fractions:

Breastfed children 6–23 months of age who had at least the minimum dietary diversity and the minimum meal frequency during the previous day/breastfed children 6–23 months of age.

Non-breastfed children 6–23 months of age who received at least two milk feedings and had at least the minimum dietary diversity not including milk feeds and the minimum meal frequency during the previous day/non-breastfed children 6–23 months of age.

Step 1: Calculate the age of the child

If the data has a variable for date of birth and date of visit, the age of the child in months can be calculated. In this dataset, the age in months has already been calculated. The next step will be to set up age categories that will make interpreting the child feeding indicators possible. This will require categorical variables for children younger than five months, children younger than 24 months and children aged 4–5 months. The data on child age in months is given in column D. Age categories can be calculated in Microsoft Excel using an IF function. Create a column and enter the formula.

$$= IF(C2 < 5, 1, 0)$$

The computer will interpret this formula as saying if the child's age (given in cell C2) is less than five months, it will be put in category 1 (younger than five months), and if the age is greater than five months, it will be put in category 0 (older than five months). This process can be repeated to calculate the rest of the age categories required.

Step 2: Calculate the first indicator: early initiation of breastfeeding

The indicator early initiation of breastfeeding describes the proportion of children younger than 24 months old, who were put to the breast within one hour of birth. Therefore, the variables required are children younger than 24 months and timing of initiation of breastfeeding. The variable for children younger than 24 months was created in the previous step. In this dataset, 0 codes for a child who was put to the breast within one hour of birth, and 1 codes for children who were put to breast after one hour after birth or not at all. This information may be obtained using a pivot table in Excel. Navigate to Insert on Excel and select pivot table. A wizard will appear, which will ask you to define the range of data to include in the table. Choose the whole range of data and opt to open a pivot table on a new sheet. You can now choose the variables to include in the pivot table. Select children younger than 24 months, and when the child put to breast as the variables for the pivot table. Move 'when child put to the breast' to the rows field, and 'sum of children younger than 24 months to the sum values field'. The total number of children is 81, of which 51 are coded '0' and 30 are coded '1'. The indicator can be calculated by dividing the number of children coded 0/total children younger than 24 months. Therefore, 62.9% of children were put to the breast within one hour of birth.

A similar procedure can be used to calculate the indicators for exclusive breastfeeding rates at different ages.

Our second worked example presents fictitious data collected at primary health facilities, and it is secondary data. Here, we use the raw data to present information that is intelligible to readers. The indicators are as follows:

1. First antenatal visit <20 weeks
2. Child underweight <2 years (new)
3. Child <5 years on food supplementation (new)
4. Infant exclusively breastfed at the third HepB dose
5. Vitamin A dose 12–59 months

One method of presenting this data is to prepare graphs. This makes it easier to make comparisons and observe trends over time. Begin by selecting the tab containing the clinical data, navigate to insert, and then create a pivot table. Select all of the data available. Place the pivot table in a new tab. Select all of the variables to include in the pivot table. Now that the pivot table has been set up, we can create an interactive chart that allows us to manipulate which data is being presented. While on the pivot table tab, select 'insert' and then insert a graph. Once the graph has been inserted, there will be options on the graph to toggle between viewing all of the clinic data, or only the rural or urban clinic, or dividing the data up by time frame.

References

Anand, S.S., Hawkes, C., De Souza, R.J. et al. (2015). Food consumption and its impact on cardiovascular disease: importance of solutions focused on the globalised food system: a report from the workshop convened by the World Heart Federation. *J. Am. Coll. Cardiol.* 66 (14): 1590–1614.

Defechereux, T., Paolucci, F., Mirelman, A. et al. (2012). Health care priority setting in Norway: a multicriteria decision analysis. *BMC Health Serv. Res.* 12 (39).

Fold, N. (2002). Lead firms and competition in 'bi-polar' commodity chains: grinders and branders in the global cocoa-chocolate industry. *J. Agrarian Change* 2 (2): 228–247.

Friedman, G. (2014). *Review of National Nutrition Surveillance Systems*. Washington, DC: FHI 360/FANTA.

Labadarios, D., Steyn, N.P., Maunder, E. et al. (2005). The National Food Consumption Survey (NFCS): South Africa, 1999. *Public Health Nutr.* 8 (5): 533–543.

Mason, J.B., Habicht, J.P., Tabatabai, H., and Valverde, V. (1984). *Nutritional Surveillance*. Geneva: World Health Organisation.

Republic of South Africa (2003). Department of Health. Government notice. No. R2003. Regulations relating to the fortification of certain foodstuffs. Section 15 (1) of the Foodstuffs, Cosmetics and Disinfectants Act, No. 54 of 1972.

Shisana, O., Labadarios, D., Rehle, T. et al. (2013). *South African National Health and Nutrition Examination Survey (SANHANES-1)*. Cape Town: HSRC Press.

Tansey, G. and Worsley, A. (1995). *The Food System*. London: Routledge.

Tuffrey, V. and Hall, A. (2016). Methods of nutritional surveillance in low-income countries. *Emerg. Themes Epidemiol.* 13 (4).

Youngkong, S., Kapiriri, L., and Baltussen, R. (2009). Setting priorities for health interventions in developing countries: A review of empirical studies. *Trop Med. Int. Health.* 14 (8): 930–939.

4 Nutrition and Infectious Disease

4.1 Introduction

Communicable diseases, also called infectious diseases, are caused by virulent or pathogenic organisms that are transmitted from host to host. Infectious diseases are a global health issue, as globalisation has made it easier to spread pathogens across borders. While infectious diseases affect high-, middle-, and low-income countries, people living in low- and middle-income countries are particularly vulnerable because of poverty, inequality, poorer access to infrastructure and greater vulnerability to disease and poor health.

4.1.1 Communicable Diseases and Non-Communicable Diseases

Communicable diseases are also called 'infectious diseases' (Sharma and Atri 2010) and are caused by *pathogenic* or *virulent* microorganisms. The pathogens that cause these diseases are transmitted between hosts, and the diseases tend to be acute (Global Burden of Disease Study 2013 Collaborators 2015). These diseases may be cured with antimicrobial medications.

Non-communicable diseases are chronic diseases, which progress slowly and endure for a long period of time (Sharma and Atri 2010). They develop from a non-contagious origin (McKenna et al. 1998), are characteristically incurable and are associated with functional impairment or disability.

Communicable diseases include food and waterborne diseases such as *Escherichia coli*, cholera and rotavirus. They may be sexually transmitted or bloodborne as in the case of human immunodeficiency virus (HIV) and hepatitis B. Tuberculosis is an example of an inhalation or respiratory tract infection. Communicable diseases such as malaria can be transmitted by vectors. Non-communicable diseases include

Nutrition and Global Health, First Edition. Shawn W. McLaren.
© 2023 John Wiley & Sons Ltd. Published 2023 by John Wiley & Sons Ltd.

cardiovascular diseases such as stroke and hypertension, neoplasms and respiratory tract diseases such as chronic obstructive pulmonary disease (COPD) and type 2 diabetes mellitus (T2DM).

4.1.1.1 Infectious Diseases and Globalisation

Globalisation affects the spread of disease. Air travel helped to facilitate the spread of SARS in 2002–2004 (Ruan et al. 2006). Infectious diseases are a *global health issue*, affecting both the developing and developed world. Infectious and communicable diseases are more common in low- and middle-income countries (Sharma and Atri 2010). This is because poverty, inequality and poorer access to infrastructure result in increased vulnerability to disease and poor health (Marmot 2005). The communicable disease burden is higher in developing countries and is intimately related to access to resources as well as nutritional status. However, the predominant form of malnutrition – overnutrition – in developed countries is now emerging as a risk factor for communicable disease, as was demonstrated by the links between raised mortality risk from COVID-19 infection amongst people with obesity.

4.2 The Relationship Between Infectious Disease and Malnutrition

Disease and malnutrition are interrelated. The UNICEF conceptual framework on malnutrition (Figure 4.1) describes disease and inadequate dietary intake as immediate causes of malnutrition and death. Underlying causes refer to inadequate access to food, care, health services and a healthy environment. Malnutrition predisposes people to a higher risk of disease, and disease can lead to malnutrition. Nutrition interventions may be nutrition specific, addressing the immediate causes of malnutrition, or nutrition sensitive, addressing the underlying causes of malnutrition.

The basic causes of malnutrition stem from the social, political and ideological superstructure of a country. Underlying causes of malnutrition include inadequate food security, inadequate care for women and children, insufficient access to health services and an unhealthy environment. These underlying causes increase the risk of inadequate dietary intake and the development of disease, and the outcomes are malnutrition and death.

The disease–malnutrition–poverty cycle describes the intergenerational nature of the relationship between these three factors (Figure 4.2). A consequence of malnutrition during childhood is impaired development and immune system function, predisposing individuals to

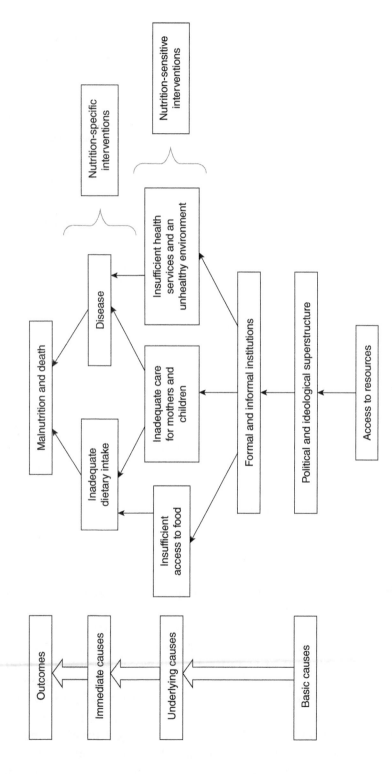

Figure 4.1: Interventions in the context of the *UNICEF Conceptual Framework on the Causes of Malnutrition* (UNICEF 1997).

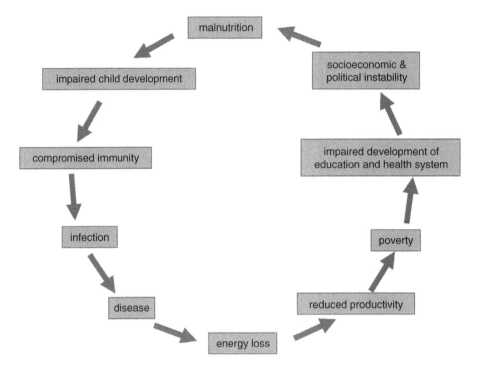

Figure 4.2: The disease–malnutrition–poverty cycle (Schaible and Kaufmann 2007/PLOS/CC BY).

disease and reduced productivity, inhibiting people from meeting their full potential and perpetuating the cycle of poor education, poverty and malnutrition (Schaible and Kaufmann 2007).

4.2.1 Nutrition-Specific Interventions

Nutrition-specific interventions address the immediate determinants of nutritional well-being. These are adequate food and nutrient intake, and are related to child feeding, caregiving and parenting practices. The aim of nutrition-specific interventions is to lower the burden of infectious disease (Ruel and Alderman 2013).

Examples of areas for nutrition-specific interventions include adolescent, preconception and maternal health and nutrition. This might involve maternal micronutrient supplementation or dietary supplementation. It may involve the promotion of optimum breast-feeding practices. Interventions that aim to prevent and manage diseases could be nutrition specific, as in the case of the treatment of acute malnutrition (Ruel and Alderman 2013). Nutrition-specific strategies that have been proven to reduce stunting prevalence include universal salt iodisation, multiple micronutrient supplementation, community-based breastfeeding and complementary feeding interventions, and community-based management of severe acute malnutrition (Haddinott et al. 2013).

4.2.2 Nutrition-Sensitive Interventions

Nutrition-sensitive interventions address the underlying determinants of nutritional well-being and development. Areas of intervention that are nutrition sensitive include food security, adequacy of caregiving resources, access to health services, and creating a safe and hygienic environment (Ruel and Alderman 2013). These areas for development include agriculture and food security, women's empowerment, water, sanitation and hygiene (WaSH), health and family planning services, and schooling (Ruel and Alderman 2013). Effective, large-scale solutions to the underlying causes of malnutrition are crucial to addressing malnutrition.

Often, the inter-relatedness of underlying causes of malnutrition is addressed concurrently by intervening in one area of a nutrition-sensitive intervention. In the example of improving access to household, school or work sanitation in an effort to lower rates of illness and infection, outcomes include improved cognitive development and ability to attend school or work (Sclar et al. 2017) (Figure 4.3). Education and household income are factors related to stunting and wasting risk (Nshimyiryo et al. 2019). By improving sanitation, other risk factors are indirectly improved, contributing to a greater overall improvement in malnutrition and mortality risk and improving lives.

Contributions to reducing stunting are comparable between nutrition-sensitive and nutrition-specific interventions, with the health and nutrition sectors as well as other sectors making important contributions

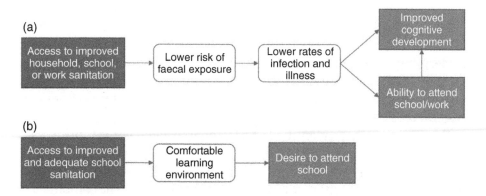

Figure 4.3: An example of addressing multiple causes of malnutrition through implementing nutrition-sensitive interventions (Sclar et al. 2017/with permission of Elsevier).

to reducing stunting (Bhutta et al. 2020). Favourable interventions from outside the nutrition sector (nutrition-sensitive interventions) include improving education amongst girls and women, reductions in fertility and wider birth spacing, and improvements in maternal and newborn care (Bhutta et al. 2020).

Successful interventions can also make use of a combination of nutrition-specific and nutrition-sensitive interventions. The Expanded Programme on Immunization (EPI) has been a very successful public health intervention since the 1970s (Wallace et al. 2012). The rotavirus vaccine is used as part of the EPI in many countries. Rotavirus is one of the leading causes of diarrhoea in children (Liu et al. 2016). Rotavirus vaccination is effective in reducing the number of episodes of severe gastroenteritis (Madhi et al. 2012), and timely vaccination has been associated with improved HAZ (Loli and Carcamo 2020) and with recovery from stunting (Faye et al. 2019).

Governments have used the EPI to deliver additional health interventions and primary care services, including distributing antihelminth chemotherapy (deworming) and nutrition-specific interventions such as vitamin A supplementation and growth monitoring and promotion. Coverage of these public health interventions is increased as the same appointments can be used to administer routine immunisations, vitamin A and deworming (Imdad et al. 2010).

Immunisation coverage is not always comprehensive and poorer, and more rural communities may be at higher risk of delayed or incomplete vaccinations (Fadnes et al. 2011). Vitamin A supplementation and deworming are recommended by the WHO for all children over the age of six months at regular six-month intervals. As children require fewer vaccinations as they get older, the opportunity to double up on these interventions with the EPI may result in fewer doses of vitamin A drops and deworming medications in older children.

A common nutrition-sensitive intervention is the provision of cash and food transfers. This is used especially in emergency settings. There is some evidence of the effectiveness of this approach to address an underlying cause of malnutrition – insufficient access to food – this form of intervention requires clear goals and actions and effective service delivery to yield successes in terms of nutritional status (Ruel and Alderman 2013).

Education has been identified as a factor associated with stunting risk. Children of parents with poor education are more likely to be stunted. In addition, stunting results in developmental delays. The education sector is therefore a good area for nutrition-sensitive intervention. The combination of early child development programmes and nutrition-sensitive interventions can be a cost-effective and efficient use of resources and result in improvements in nutritional status (Ruel and Alderman 2013).

Actions to enhance nutrition sensitivity (Ruel and Alderman 2013)

Improved targeting

Stimulate participation

Strengthen nutrition goals and actions

Optimise women's nutrition and empowerment

Nutrition-sensitive interventions are valuable and can be implemented on a large scale, addressing the underlying causes of malnutrition, as well as some of the consequences of malnutrition including impaired developmental potential (Ruel and Alderman 2013).

4.3 WaSH and Diarrhoeal Disease

This section discusses the relationship between the causes of diarrhoeal diseases, malabsorption, and malnutrition and failure to thrive. It discusses strategies to address these issues including WaSH strategies as nutrition-sensitive interventions.

4.3.1 Water

'Water is essential to sustain life, and a satisfactory (adequate, safe and accessible) supply must be available to all. Improving access to safe drinking-water can result in tangible benefits to health. Every effort should be made to achieve drinking-water that is as safe as practicable' (WHO 2017).

Drinking water describes more than just water used for drinking but also used for domestic purposes, cooking and personal hygiene. For drinking water to be considered safe, it must meet microbiological and chemical standards for drinking-water quality. Guidance on these standards is provided by the WHO Drinking-water Quality Guidelines (WHO 2017). Microbial risks to safe drinking water are largely related to exposure to faecal contamination from human and animal populations, including birds. Faeces contains a wide array of microbial pathogens, including bacteria, viruses, protozoa and helminths. Chemical contamination of water can lead to adverse health outcomes over a more prolonged period of exposure and can affect the sensory qualities of drinking water in terms of taste, colour and smell, affecting intake.

The WHO recommends that access to safe drinking water is measured by the percentage of the population using improved drinking-water sources. Improved drinking-water sources are those that protect water from outside contamination by the nature of their construction. It is important in this definition that improved water is protected from faecal matter. In nutrition and health surveys of populations, access to safe drinking water is estimated using indicators such as the proportion of the population using improved drinking-water sources. Improved drinking-water sources are on-premises piped drinking-water connections, including running water in dwellings, yards or on the plot. Improved sources also include public stand-pipes, boreholes, protected dug wells, protected springs and rainwater collection. Unimproved drinking-water sources include unprotected wells, unprotected springs, surface water from rivers, dams, lakes, ponds, streams, canals or irrigation channels, vendor-provided water delivered by tanker trucks or carts with a small tank, and bottled water. When households use another improved water source for cooking and personal hygiene, bottled water may be considered an improved water source for drinking.

4.3.2 Sanitation

Like improved water, improved sanitation refers to sanitation facilities that hygienically separate human faeces and urine from human contact. In health surveys, access to improved sanitation is measured as the proportion of people using these facilities. Improved sanitation facilities include those connected to a sewer system, septic tanks, pour-flush latrines, ventilated improved pit latrines and pit latrines with a slab or covered pit. If one or two households share access to any of these types of toilets, they are still considered improved sanitation facilities. However, if more than two households share access, they are no longer considered improved sanitation facilities. This includes public toilet facilities. Unimproved sanitation facilities do not adequately ensure that human waste is separated from human contact, and these include pit latrines without slabs and open pits. Other common examples from developing regions are hanging latrines and bucket latrines. Many people still practice open defecation in fields, forests, bodies of water or disposal of human faeces with other forms of solid waste (WHO 2017).

Worldwide, diarrhoea is one of the leading causes of death amongst children younger than five years old (Bryce et al. 2005). There is widespread carriage of pathogens in developing countries. Rotavirus, *Cryptosporidium*, *Shigella* and enterotoxigenic *E. coli* produce heat-stable toxins and are mainly responsible for diarrhoea amongst African and Asian children (Kotloff et al. 2013). Potential pathogens were identified in 83% of children with diarrhoea and 72% of controls (Kotloff et al. 2013). Rotavirus infection is a significant contributor to the incidence of diarrhoea in children younger than five years (Tate et al. 2016). Diarrhoeal diseases are closely related to childhood malnutrition, and each episode of diarrhoea that a child experiences increases their risk of malnutrition. The adjusted odds of stunting increased by 1.13 for every five diarrhoeal episodes in a pooled longitudinal study (95% CI 1.07–1.19) (Checkley et al. 2008). Diarrhoea increased the likelihood of stunting amongst Libyan children (OR = 1.58, 95% CI 1.09, 2.29) (Taguri et al. 2009). An estimated 165 million children under the age of five were stunted in 2014 (UNICEF et al. 2015). Diarrhoeal disease caused by pathogens results in poorer absorption of nutrients. Acute diarrhoeal episodes in infants are caused by mixed feeding practices and improper weaning practices (Lamberti et al. 2011). As diarrhoea and enteric infections cause malabsorption of nutrients and damage to the intestinal mucosa, Guerrant et al. (2013) have estimated that diarrhoea contributes to 43% of stunted growth seen amongst children.

Nutrient malabsorption leads to stunted growth and an associated developmental delay, disruption of immune function and a higher risk of illness and death. These are all contributing factors to the disease–malnutrition–poverty cycle. In addition to stunted growth, gastrointestinal infections from pathogens such as *Shigella* or *Salmonella* can cause blood loss and, in rare occurrences, haemolysis (Jonker et al. 2017). Schistosomiasis and protozoan infections are common in areas of poor sanitation, causing diarrhoea and blood loss (Hechenbleikner and McQuade 2015). In addition to blood loss, enteric infections can contribute to the development of anaemia as inflammation and infection promote the production of hepcidin. Hepcidin is an iron-regulating hormone that prevents iron absorbed into the duodenal cells from entering circulation. Inflammatory cytokines, including IFN-gamma, TNF-alpha and IL-6, produced during times of infection, downregulate erythropoiesis and the production of new red blood cells. The effects of diarrhoeal disease on nutrient absorption are presented in Figure 4.4.

4.4 HIV, Malaria, Tuberculosis and Intestinal Parasites

Respiratory infections, malaria, HIV and TB are responsible for high mortality rates in low- and middle-income countries. Each of these diseases has implications for nutritional status, and nutritional treatment is often integrated into strategies to address these issues.

4.4.1 HIV and AIDS

Acquired immunodeficiency syndrome (AIDS) is caused by HIV and is characterised by a weakened or depleted immune system. HIV targets a specific type of immune cell known as CD4 T-cells and replicates within these cells. There are two strains of HIV, known as HIV1 and HIV2.

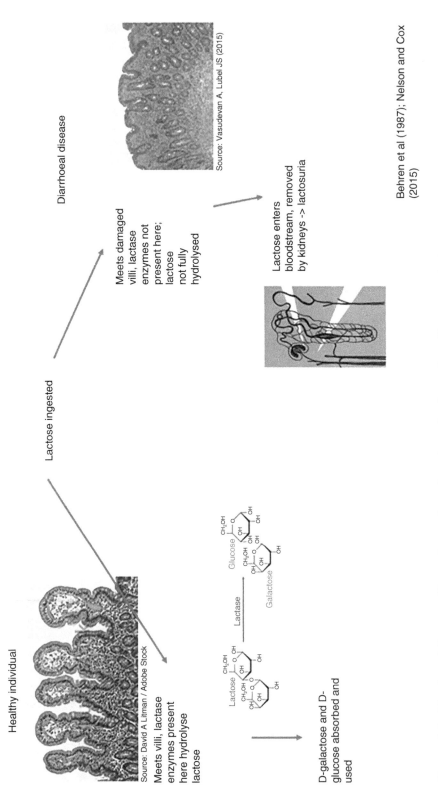

Healthy individual

Source: David A Litman / Adobe Stock

Meets villi, lactase enzymes present here hydrolyse lactose

Lactose ingested

Diarrhoeal disease

Source: Vasudevan A, Lubel JS (2015)

Meets damaged villi, lactase enzymes not present here; lactose not fully hydrolysed

Lactose enters bloodstream, removed by kidneys -> lactosuria

Behren et al (1987); Nelson and Cox (2015)

Lactose

Lactase

Glucose

Galactose

D-galactose and D-glucose absorbed and used

Figure 4.4: Diarrhoeal disease affects absorption of nutrients by damaging villous morphology.

Source: Adapted from Behren et al. 1987 and Nelson and Cox 2015.

HIV1 is thought to have broken the 'species barrier' between simians and humans between the 1880s and 1920s, with HIV2 appearing in humans in the 1940s (Wertheim and Worobey 2009). Globalisation in latter half of the twentieth century facilitated the exponential spread of the virus. HIV and AIDS is truly a global health issue.

AIDS-related deaths totalled 1.7 million worldwide in 2011 (UNAIDS 2012). Sub-Saharan Africa has been particularly affected by HIV and AIDS. According to UNAIDS (2012), there are 6 100 000 people living with HIV in South Africa. Of these, 410 000 were children under the age of 14 years. Despite the effective roll out of antiretroviral therapy (ART), 8255 people died due to AIDS in South Africa in 2011 (Statistics South Africa 2014).

HIV progresses to symptomatic AIDS when the host's immune system is depleted by interactions with the HI virus (Lackner et al. 2009). HIV primarily targets T-cell lymphocytes in the host's mucosal organ systems. This makes people living with HIV and AIDS extremely susceptible to opportunistic infections such as tuberculosis, pneumonia and gastroenteritis (Solomon et al. 2018). According to Kimani-Murage (2013), HIV has a significant effect on nutritional outcomes in children. There was a strong association between HIV and HAZ as well as WAZ in multiple regression models (Kimani-Murage 2013). The authors reported that the number of HIV-positive children in the study receiving ART was negligible. According to this study, mean values for HAZ, WAZ and WHZ were significantly lower ($p < 0.05$) in HIV-infected children than non-infected children (Kimani-Murage 2013).

HIV is transmitted via mucous membranes. It is transmitted through sexual intercourse and contact with infected secretions. Vertical transmission, known as mother to child transmission (MTCT), can occur in utero, during labour or through breastfeeding, and many strategies to reduce the spread of HIV have focused on prevention of mother to child transmission (PMTCT). HIV can also be transmitted by contact with infected bodily fluids and occurs as a result of needle-stick injuries or sharing needles (Pribram 2011). The mode of transmission of HIV has led to widespread fear and stigma surrounding the condition (Whiteside 2016).

4.4.1.1 Targeting Interventions

Very seldom HIV status alone used to target strategies (de Menezes and Ogden 2011). Difficulties arise from stigma and social disharmony. Targeting the chronically sick or poor as proxies could result in those being labelled as HIV positive. Therefore, community engagement is an important aspect of HIV interventions. Potential target groups for nutritional interventions include communities with high HIV prevalence, people using HIV services, child-headed households, HIV-positive pregnant women, and infants and young children of HIV-positive mothers.

Nutrition interventions related to HIV and AIDS need to be related to a specific outcome. In the case of targeted food supplementation schemes, the aim is to support food insecure households. This type of intervention attempts to prevent malnutrition. Therapeutic feeding is a strategy to address existing malnutrition, in order to improve the immune response and reduce the mortality risk and is often used as a strategy in conjunction with ART. Providing supplementary food or therapeutic feeding can also be used as a strategy to improve adherence to HIV and TB treatment. School-feeding schemes can make an indirect contribution to reducing the effects of HIV and poor food security. Food has also been used as an incentive for attendance at PMTCT events.

Improved access to treatment in the form of medication, support, and appropriate nutrition and effective implementation of prevention strategies including condoms or male circumcision help to reduce the risk of malnutrition amongst HIV-positive people. These strategies also result in improvements in life expectancy and reduction in AIDS-related mortality. However, there is potentially a large societal impact; people live longer but require care, costly medications and suffer disabilities associated with HIV and AIDS.

4.4.1.2 Antiretroviral Medications (ARVs)

ARVs transformed HIV/AIDS from progressive, terminal illness to chronic, manageable disease. There are six classes of ARV drugs working at different stages of the HIV life cycle. Some of these medications are associated with adverse effects, food–drug reactions and drug–drug reactions. Adherence to treatment is extremely important.

Although HIV has a negative effect on child growth, access to anti-retroviral medication improves the growth of HIV-infected children. A study on malnourished (WAZ, WHZ or HAZ < -2) HIV-positive children showed that significant catch-up growth occurred in the 24 months following initiation onto ART (Jesson et al. 2015). Nevaripine prophylaxis has been shown to significantly reduce the wasting prevalence amongst HIV-exposed as well as HIV-positive infants within the first year of life (Ram et al. 2012). ART appears to have a positive effect on growth outcomes in infants and is related to the timing of infection and initiation onto ART (Ram et al. 2012).

4.4.1.3 HIV and Malnutrition

Malnutrition may occur at any stage of the disease. It is the result of reduced food intake, malabsorption and hypermetabolism. Poor nutritional status is associated with disease progression, morbidity and mortality (Kotler et al. 1989; Wheeler et al. 1998).

HIV has a significant impact on the gastrointestinal tract, and it has implications for nutritional status. The gut plays a fundamental role in maintaining nutritional status as it absorbs nutrients from food. The gut also plays an important role in immune function, protecting the body from pathogens from the diet. Both of these functions rely on the mucosal barrier in the gastrointestinal tract. Simultaneously, the gut is home to a diverse microbiota, species of which can be beneficial in some regions of the gut but harmful in others when bacterial translocation occurs. The immune function of the gut is enhanced by the presence of a very high concentration of immune cells. As HIV affects mucosal membranes and immune cells, the gastrointestinal system presents a significant target for HIV (Ahluwalia et al. 2017). An increased rate of immune activation and inflammation because of HIV infection disrupts mucosal repair in the gut and results in enteropathy (Dandekar 2007). This is a cause of persistent diarrhoea in seropositive people and can be the first indication of HIV infection (Miller et al. 2008). Damage to the intestinal mucosa and villi results in poorer nutrient absorption, which is a mechanism involved in malnutrition in HIV.

In addition, ART may affect erythropoiesis (Redig and Berliner 2013). Viruses are also known to directly affect erythropoiesis (Morinet et al. 2017).

4.4.1.4 Breastfeeding and HIV

Breastfeeding is associated with vertical transmission risk and was a controversial area of nutrition during the first decades of HIV treatment strategy. Prior to the availability of ART, researchers questioned the effect of exclusive breastfeeding (EBF), formula feeding and mixed feeding practices on HIV transmission. Doherty et al. (2006) documented uncertainty about the safety of breastfeeding amongst HIV-positive women. It is now known that the MTCT rate is similar for exclusive breastfed and exclusive formula-fed infants. Exclusive breastfeeding or exclusive formula feeding are favourable to mixed feeding (Coutsoudis et al. 1999). Cultural norms that are not conducive to breastfeeding, including the introduction of fluids and foods other than breastmilk as early as three months, were fed by the stigma and uncertainty attached to HIV (Doherty et al. 2006). Mixed feeding, early introduction of complementary foods and choosing breastmilk substitutes have a negative impact on child growth and HIV infection risk. Findings like this aided in forming infant feeding recommendations for HIV-positive women, which included exclusive breastfeeding. Improved community-based support for ART and increased coverage of child feeding information could aid in reducing vertical transmission of HIV and improve the growth of infants and young children. Breastfeeding is safe with low viral load, resulting from ART use. The HIV epidemic had an impact on child feeding practices. Widespread antiretroviral medication only became available in the mid-2000s. Community-based support for HIV-positive pregnant women increased the likelihood of initiating ART during pregnancy (Fatti et al. 2016). Improved community-based support for ART and increased coverage of child feeding information could aid in reducing vertical transmission of HIV and improve the growth of infants and young children.

4.4.2 Malaria

There has been an improvement in the incidence of malaria worldwide; however, it is still a significant public health concern that impacts nutritional status. The number of cases of malaria decreased from 251 million cases in 2010 to 228 million cases in 2018. However, the rate of reduction has slowed over this time period. Africa, Southeast Asia and the Eastern Mediterranean have high rates of malaria, with 93% of all cases occurring in the African region. Malaria was a cause of 405 000 deaths in 2018. Children younger than five years of age are particularly vulnerable, and two-thirds of malaria deaths are amongst children. Malaria infection during pregnancy is a significant contributor to low birthweight risk amongst infants. Eleven million pregnant women were exposed to malaria in 2019, resulting in more than 800 000 low birthweight infants. Pregnant women in sub-Saharan Africa are at a particularly high risk of exposure (WHO 2019).

Malaria is caused by the plasmodium virus. *P. falciparum* is the most virulent malaria-causing species and is the cause of almost all malaria cases in sub-Saharan Africa (WHO 2000). The plasmodium life cycle begins when an infected mosquito bites a human and takes blood, injecting sporozoites into the tissues. Sporozoites then travel to the liver, infecting cells and forming schizonts – cells containing developing trophozoites. When the schizonts rupture, trophozoites are released. These enter the erythrocytes, replicating viral RNA and forming erythrocytic schizonts. The schizonts rupture, releasing sporozoites. Immature trophozoites may form gametocytes. Mosquitoes biting infected people to obtain a blood meal pick up erythrocytes containing gametocytes that will develop into sporozoites within the mosquito, which can then be transmitted to other people.

As the plasmodium life cycle involves red blood cells, malaria impacts iron status through a combination of haemolysis, erythrocyte sequestration and impaired erythropoiesis (Abdulkareem et al. 2017). Severe anaemia and malaria amongst children are often inter-related, with almost 2 million of 24 million children infected with *P. falciparum* presenting with severe anaemia in sub-Saharan Africa (WHO 2019 World Malaria Report).

Malaria infection is common amongst children admitted to the hospital with SAM. Poor height gain during recovery was observed amongst children admitted to the hospital with SAM with malaria (Oldenburg et al. 2018). Mosquitoes are the vector which are responsible for transmitting malaria.

Malaria risk is higher amongst children whose households collect water from open sources such as rivers or streams (non-improved sources) (Teh et al. 2018). Teh et al. (2018) found that malaria risk was highest amongst children aged 5–9 years, while the risk of malnutrition was highest amongst children before the 5th birthday near Mount Cameroon. However, Gone et al. (2017) found that plasmodium exposure before the age of five years was a risk factor for malnutrition. Clinical malaria is associated with malnutrition amongst children, and malnutrition is an important factor in malaria-associated morbidity (Ehrhardt et al. 2006). Effective large-scale malaria prevention programmes need to be integrated with nutrition programmes to achieve the desired outcomes (Ehrhardt et al. 2006).

4.4.3 Tuberculosis (TB)

Tuberculosis is a disease caused by the pathogenic bacterium *Mycobacterium tuberculosis*. TB is a pulmonary disease but can also affect bone, the central nervous system and other organ systems (Smith 2003). *Mycobacterium tuberculosis* bacilli are transmitted to the lungs through inhalation of aerosol droplets. Once bacilli enter the lungs, macrophages found in the pulmonary tissue engulf them as part of the normal immune response. The host immune system determines how the disease progresses once it has taken place (Smith 2003). Genetics of the host immune system as well as nutritional status and physiological state are factors that will play a role in the outcome (Smith 2003). If the host's immune system is unable to destroy the bacilli, the bacilli will proliferate and the macrophage will burst, releasing more bacilli. Approximately a week after initial infection, if the immune system is overwhelmed in the initial stage, the TB bacilli will begin to reproduce exponentially. This exponential increase in bacterial cells will continue for approximately two weeks, until more immune cells enter the lungs, and the number of new bacilli is balanced with the number destroyed by macrophages. The majority of people with TB infection will be asymptomatic after this stage. The bacilli and infected macrophages are encased in a complex known as a Ghon focus, which prevents further spread of the disease and results in the infected person no longer being contagious once the Ghon focus has calcified. During this stage, TB can infect the lymph nodes, resulting in a Ghon complex. The bacilli can survive for years in the infected macrophages contained in the Ghon focus. In a small proportion of people with TB, the TB may become re-activated and progress to symptomatic TB, which is transmissible and causes the symptoms associated with TB including coughing.

The incidence rate of TB infection is declining by about 2% per year (WHO 2019). However, in 2018, 1.5 million adults died globally from TB, and the disease is one of the 10 leading causes of death caused by an infectious agent (WHO 2019). Additionally, 1.1 million children contracted TB and 205 000 child deaths were attributed to this disease in 2018 (WHO 2019). Ending the TB epidemic by 2030 is one of the health targets of the Sustainable Development Goals. The WHO's End TB Strategy aims to reduce the number of new cases of TB by 80%, the number of TB deaths by 90% and protecting all families affected by TB from catastrophic costs by 2030.

4.4.3.1 TB in Children

Children's exposure to TB is affected by the prevalence of TB in their community, population structure and housing structures (Seddon and Shingadia 2014). The child's age and interaction with the community influence the level of exposure to TB (Seddon and Shingadia 2014). Alcohol intake in the community is another factor (Seddon and Shingadia 2014). TB amongst children and adolescents can be more difficult to diagnose and treat in resource-poor environments. A lack of resources in sub-Saharan Africa also impacts the accuracy of TB prevalence and incidence in this region (Seddon and Shingadia 2014). Berman et al. (1992) found that half of children diagnosed with TB during their study had not been previously diagnosed with TB, indicating that children are often missed.

4.4.3.2 TB and Nutritional Status

TB infection contributes directly and indirectly to malnutrition (Collins et al. 2006). Symptomatic TB results in fatigue, weakness, shortness of breath, chest pain and fever. As a result of these symptoms, adults with active TB infection have difficulty continuing work and lose financial opportunities. The physical weakness that is associated with active TB means that labour-intensive work including subsistence agriculture is problematic. These indirect effects of TB on livelihoods and food security also contribute to childhood malnutrition (Collins et al. 2006).

A large proportion of people with TB are concurrently anaemic (Minchella et al. 2015). The anaemia associated with TB may be either iron-responsive due to simple iron deficiency or the anaemia may be a result of the TB infection, caused by immune activation and inflammation (Minchella et al. 2015). Evidence suggests that anaemia resulting from inflammation resolves with TB treatment, and anaemia resulting from iron deficiency or a combination of iron deficiency and inflammation requires further nutrition intervention (Minchella et al. 2015).

Vitamin B6, also called pyridoxine, is involved in red blood cell metabolism, nervous and immune system function and converting tryptophan to niacin. It is a co-enzyme in amino acid metabolic pathways and is involved in blood glucose homeostasis. Deficiency results in sleepiness, fatigue, cheilosis, glossitis, stomatitis in adults, abnormal

EEGs and seizures. Isoniazid, a drug commonly used to treat TB, competitively inhibits pyridoxine's metabolic roles (Snider 1980). Therefore, pyridoxine supplementation is recommended in people taking this drug for TB treatment to prevent symptoms of deficiency.

4.4.3.3 TB Treatment

Patients with TB respond well to treatment, with a good prognosis for patients who receive timely and appropriate treatment. Delayed diagnosis is potentially extremely dangerous, particularly in children, due to the risk of tuberculosis meningitis (Marais and Schaaf 2014).

An important challenge in treating TB and preventing mortality from this infectious disease is the emergence of multidrug resistant TB (MDR-TB). The WHO has estimated that half a million cases of TB are resistant to rifampicin, which is considered the most effective first-line drug. Therefore, adherence to medication is extremely important to prevent the development of drug-resistant strains of the pathogen (Table 4.1).

Table 4.1: Summary of the first-line TB drugs and dosage recommendations in children.

First-line drugs	Mode and mechanism of action	Main toxicities
Isoniazid (INH)	Bactericidal – inhibits cell wall synthesis; most potent early bactericidal activity offering the best protection to companion drugs Contributes mainly by rapidly killing actively metabolising extracellular bacilli; contributes to sterilisation if given for a prolonged period	Hepatitis; peripheral neuropathy
Rifampicin (RMP)	Bactericidal and sterilising – inhibits RNA synthesis; contributes by killing extracellular and slower growing intracellular bacilli; important contribution to sterilisation	Hepatitis; orange discoloration of secretions; drug–drug interactions
Pyrazinamide (PZA)	Sterilising – disrupts energy metabolism; contributes by specifically killing bacilli that persist within the acidic centres of caseating granulomas	Hepatitis; arthralgia
Ethambutol (EMB)	Bacteriostatic – inhibits cell wall synthesis; contributes mainly by offering some additional protection against drug-resistant mutants	Visual disturbance (acuity, colour vision)

Source: Adapted from Marais and Schaaf 2014.

4.4.4 Parasites and Helminths

Helminths are common parasites of the human gastrointestinal tract. The main categories of helminths are nematodes (roundworms), trematodes (flatworms) and cestodes (tapeworms) (Keo et al. 2015).

Helminths enter the human gastrointestinal tract through ingestion of fertilised helminth eggs. Exposure to contaminated soil or water, or food which has been contaminated with helminth eggs, can result in helminth infestation (Gupta et al. 2009). Infants and young children exploring their environment by chewing or transferring objects and soil to their mouths may pick up helminth eggs. Vegetables that have not been adequately washed before consumption can be a route of entry in children and adults.

Infestation is associated with malnutrition in children and is commonly found in the gastrointestinal tracts of children with severe acute malnutrition (Burzigi and Uganda 2015). Consequences of helminth infection include intestinal bleeding, leading to anaemia, nutrient malabsorption, diarrhoea and reduced appetite (Taylor-Robinson et al. 2019). According to Awasthi and Bundy (2007), hookworms can cause blood losses of up to 100 ml per day. Hookworms are amongst the most common species of helminth found in children, followed by *Giadia lamblia*. *G. lamblia* is associated with a high risk of diarrhoea (Burzigi and Uganda 2015).

Helminth infections are commonly treated with medications including mebendazole or albendazole. WHO protocols recommend that children receive periodic treatment with these medications regardless of diagnosis as a treatment and prevention measure. However, there has been evidence that a single dose of mebendazole has no effect on child growth (Joseph et al. 2015). A possible explanation for the lack of effect of antihelminth chemotherapy on nutritional status amongst children is the high rates of re-infection in areas endemic with helminths (Adegnika et al. 2014). Therefore, complementary strategies such as improved WaSH interventions play an important role in prevention. Washing raw vegetables before consuming them has been shown to be an effective method of removing helminth eggs (Avcioglu et al. 2011).

4.5 Integrated Management of Childhood Illness (IMCI)

IMCI is an integrated approach to childhood illness that aims to reduce the number of child deaths globally by improving case management skills of healthcare staff, improving overall health systems and family and community practices.

IMCI is a widely implemented global health strategy, which has been adopted by 102 countries worldwide. The IMCI model was developed in 1995 to deliver primary healthcare services to children younger than five years of age. IMCI was developed from the recognition that there are many interrelated factors that impact childhood illness and mortality risk, and that children may display overlapping signs of illness. Therefore, the severity of illness is the primary concern instead of a specific diagnosis. An important underlying concept for IMCI is that communicable diseases including pneumonia, malaria, diarrhoea and measles as well as malnutrition are implicated in the majority of preventable under-five child deaths. The strategy makes use of both preventative and curative approaches to reduce the burden of disease amongst children younger than five years of age.

The three main components of IMCI are as follows:

- Improving skills of health workers
- Strengthening health services
- Improving family and community practices

4.5.1 Implementation

Children younger than five years are assessed at primary healthcare facilities using the IMCI danger signs. Danger signs include the following:

- Child unable to drink or breastfeed
- Child is vomiting everything
- Child has had convulsions
- Child is lethargic or unconscious

Children who display any of the danger signs should be referred to a hospital for immediate treatment. It is good practice to identify children displaying these signs in queues in primary health facilities to triage them for immediate assessment and appropriate referral. Timing is important as these children may deteriorate rapidly and are at a high risk of mortality. It is important that healthcare workers ask caregivers about children displaying the danger signs as they may not be immediately apparent on observation.

Child feeding is covered by IMCI. Practitioners should offer advice on appropriate feeding for the child's age. An assessment of child feeding should be included as part of the IMCI assessment of the child. This is particularly important amongst children younger than two years of age and those showing anthropometric deficits on their growth charts. Questions that could be asked by health workers should focus on the following:

- If the child is being breastfed.
- How often the child is breastfed?
- If breastfeeding also takes place at night.
- If the child has any other food or fluids and how often.
- How is the child fed and by whom?

Pandya et al. (2018) identified barriers to the effective implementation of IMCI. These include fragmented programmes within the IMCI, ineffective staff and high levels of staff rotation. Approaches to improve the implementation of IMCI include using standardised health records, which include IMCI activities, as well as careful monitoring and practice audit (Pandya et al. 2018).

References

Abdulkareem, B.O., Adam, A.O., Ahmed, A.O. et al. (2017). Malaria-induced anaemia and sérum micronutrientes in asymptomatic Plasmodium falciparum infected patients. *J. Parasit. Dis.* 41: 1093–1097.

Adegnika, A.A., Zinsou, J.F., Issifou, S. et al. (2014). Randomised, controlled, assessor-blind clinical trial to assess the efficacy of single- versus repeated-dose albendazole to treat *Ascaris lumbricoides*, *Trichuris trichiura*, and hookworm infection. *Antimicrob. Agents Chemother.* 58 (5): 2535–2540.

Ahluwalia, B., Magnussen, M.K., and Ohman, L. (2017). Mucosal immune system of the gastrointestinal tract: maintaining balance between the good and the bad. *Scand. J. Gastroenterol.* 52 (11): 1185–1193.

Avcioglu, H., Soykan, E., and Tarakci, U. (2011). Control of helminth contamination or raw vegetables by washing. *Vector-borne Zoonotic Dis.* 11 (2): 189–191.

Awasthi, S. and Bundy, A. (2007). Intestinal nematode infection and anaemia in developing countries. *BMJ* 334: 1064.

Behrens, R.H., Lunn, P.G., Northrop, C.A. et al. (1987). Factors affecting the integrity of the intestinal mucosa of Gambian children. *Am. J. Clin. Nutr.* 45 (6): 1433–1441.

Berman, S., Kibel, M.A., Fourie, P.B., and Strebel, P.M. (1992). Childhood tuberculosis and tuberculosis meningitis: High incidence rates in the Western Cape of South Africa. *Tuber. Lung Dis.* 73 (6): 349–355.

Bhutta, Z.A., Askeer, N., Keats, E.C. et al. (2020). How countries can reduce child stunting at scale: lessons from exemplar studies. *Am. J. Clin. Nutr.* 112 (S2): 894S–904S.

Bryce, J., Boschi-Pinto, C., Shibuya, K., and Black, R.E. (2005). WHO estimates of the causes of death in children. *Lancet* 365: 1147–1152.

Burzigi, E. and Uganda, K. (2015). Prevalence of intestinal parasites, and its association with severe acute malnutrition related diarrhoea. *J. Biol. Agric. Healthcare* 5 (2): 81–91.

Checkley, W., Buckley, G., Gilman, R.H. et al. (2008). Multi-country analysis of the effects of diarrhoea on childhood stunting. *Int. J. Epidemiol.* 37 (4): 816–830. https://doi.org/10.1093/ije/dyn099.

Collins, S., Sadler, K., Dent, N. et al. (2006). Key issues in the success of community-based management of severe malnutrition. *Food Nutr. Bull.* 27 (S3): S49–S82.

Constantini, A., Guiliodoro, S., Butini, L. et al. (2009). Abnormalities of erythropoeisis during HIV-1 disease: A longitudinal analysis. *J. Acquir. Immune Defic. Syndr.* 52 (1): 70–74.

Coutsoudis, A., Kubendran, P., Spooner, E. et al. (1999). Influence of infant-feeding patterns in early mother-to-child transmission of HIV-1 in Durban, South Africa: a prospective cohort study. *Lancet* 354 (9177): 471–476.

Dandekar, S. (2007). Pathogenesis of HIV in the gastrointestinal tract. *Curr. HIV/AIDS Rep.* 4: 10–15.

De Menezes, C. and Ogden, K. (2011). Community in resource-limited settings. Found in Pribram V (Ed). *Nutrition and HIV.* Wiley-Blackwell, United Kingdom.

Doherty, T., Chopra, M., Nkonki, L. et al. (2006). Effect of HIV epidemic on infant feeding in South Africa: 'when they see me coming withthe tins they laugh at me'. *Bull. World Health Organ.* 84 (2).

Ehrhardt, S., Burchard, G.D., Mantel, C. et al. (2006). Malaria, anaemia, and malnutrition in African children-defining intervention priorities. *J. Infect. Dis.* 194 (1): 108–114.

Fadnes, L.T., Jackson, D., Engebretsen, I.M.S. et al. (2011). Vaccination coverage and timeliness in three South African areas: A prospective study. *BMC Public Health* 11 (404).

Fatti, G., Shaikh, N., Eley, B., and Grimwood, A. (2016). Effectiveness of community-based support for pregnant women living with HIV: a cohort study in South Africa. *AIDS Care* 28 (S1): 114–118.

Faye, C.M., Fonn, S., and Levin, J. (2019). Factors associated with recovery from stunting among under-five children in two Nairobi informal settlements. *PLoS One* 14 (4): e0215488.

Global Burden of Disease 2013 Study Collaborators (2015). Global, regional, and national incidence, prevalence and years lived with disability for 301 acute and chronic diseases and injuries in 188 countries, 1990-2013: a systematic analysis for the Global Burden of Disease Study 2013. *Lancet* 386: 743–800.

Gone, T., Lemango, F., Eliso, E. et al. (2017). The association between malaria and malnutrition among under-five children in Shashogo District, Southern Ethiopia: a case control study. *Infect. Dis. Poverty* 6 (1): 9.

Guerrant, R.L., DeBoer, M.D., Moore, S.R. et al. (2013). The impoverished gut- a triple burden of diarrhoea, stunting and chronic disease. *Nat. Rev. Gastroenterol. Hepatol.* 10: 220–229.

Gupta, N., Khan, D.K., and Santra, S.C. (2009). Prevalence of intestinal helminth eggs on vegetables grown in wastewater-irrigated areas of Titagarh, West Bengal, India. *Food Control* 20 (10): 942–945.

Haddinott, J., Alderman, H., Behrman, J.R. et al. (2013). The economic rationale for investing in stunting reduction. *Matern. Child Nutr.* 9 (S2): 69–82.

Hechenbleikner, E.M. and McQuade, J.A. (2015). Parasitic colitis. *Clin. Colon Rectal Surg.* 28 (2): 79–86.

Imdad, A., Herzer, K., Mayo-Wilson, E. et al. (2010). Vitamin A supplementation for preventing morbidity and mortality in children from 6 months to 5 years of age. *Cochrane Database Syst. Rev.* 12 (CD008524): https://doi.org/10.1002/14651858.CD008524.pub2.

Jesson, J., Masson, D., Adonon, A. et al. (2015). Prevalence of malnutrition among HIV-infected children in central and west African HIV-care programmes supported by the Growing Up Programme in 2011: A cross-sectional study. *BMC Infect. Dis.* 15: 216.

Jonker, F.A.M., te Poel, E., Bates, I., and van Hensbroek, M.B. (2017). Anaemia, iron deficiency and susceptibility to infection in children in sub-Saharan Africa, guideline dilemmas. *Br. J. Haematol.* 177 (6): 878–883.

Joseph, S.A., Casapía, M., Montresor, A. et al. (2015). The effect of deworming on growth in one-year-old children living in a soil-transmitted helminth-endemic area of peru: a randomized controlled trial. *PLoS Negl. Trop. Dis.* 9 (10): e0004020. https://doi.org/10.1371/journal.pntd.0004020.

Keo, T., Leung, J., and Weisntock, J.V. (2015). *Parasitic diseases: Helminths. In Yamada's Textbook of Gastroenterology* (ed. Podolsky et al.), 2337–2377. John Wiley and Sons.

Kimani-Murage, and E.W. (2013). Exploring the paradox: Double burden of malnutrition in rural South Africa. *Glob. Health Action* 6: https://doi.org/10.3402/gha.v6i0.19249.

Kotler, D., Tiery, A., Wang, J., and Pierson, R. (1989). Magnitude of body-cell mass depletion and timing of death from wasting in AIDS. *Am. J. Clin. Nutr.* 50: 444–447.

Kotloff, K.L., Nataro, J.P., Blackwelder, W.C. et al. (2013). Burden and aetiology of diarrhoeal disease in infants and young children in developing countries (the Global Enteric Multicenter Study, GEMS): a prospective, case-control study. *Lancet* 382: 209–222.

Lackner, A.A., Mohan, M., and Veazy, R.S. (2009). The gastrointestinal tract and AIDS pathogenesis. *Gostroenterology* 136 (6): 1966–1978.

Lamberti, L.M., Fischer Walker, C.L., Noiman, A. et al. (2011). Breastfeeding and the risk for diarrhea morbidity and mortality. *BMC Public Health* 11 (S15): S3–S15.

Liu, J., Platts-Mills, J.A., Juma, J. et al. (2016). Use of quantitative molecular diagnostic methods to identify causes of diarrhoea in children: a reanalysis of the GEMS case-control study. *Lancet* 388 (10051): 1291–1301.

Loli, S. and Carcamo, C.P. (2020). Rotavirus vaccination and stunting: Secondary data analysis from the Peruvian Demographic and Health Survey. *Vaccine* 38 (50): 8010–8015.

Madhi, S.A., Kirsten, M., Louw, C. et al. (2012). Efficacy and immunogenicity of two or three dose rotavirus-vaccine regimen in South African children over two consecutive rotavirus-seasons: a randomized, double-blind, placebo-controlled trial. *Vaccine* 27 (30 Suppl 1): A44–A51. https://doi.org/10.1016/j.vaccine.2011.08.080. PMID: 22520136.

Marais, B.J. and Schaaf, H.S. (2014). Tuberculosis in children. *Cold Spring Harb. Perspect. Med.* 4 (9): a017855.

Marmot, M. (2005). Social determinants of health inequalities. *Lancet* 365 (9464): 1099–1104.

McKenna, M.T., Taylor, W.R., Marks, J.S., and Koplan, J.P. (1998). Current issues and challenges in chronic disease control. In: *Chronic Disease Epidemiology and Control*, 2e (ed. R.C. Brownson, P.L. Remington and J.R. Davis). Washington, DC: American Public Health Association.

Miller, T.L., Agostoni, C., Duggan, C. et al. (2008). Gastrointestinal and nutritional complications of human immunodeficiency virus infection. *J. Paediatr. Gastroenterol. Nutr.* 47: 247–253.

Minchella, P.A., Donkor, S., Owolabi, O. et al. (2015). Complex anaemia in tuberculosis: the need to consider causes and timing when designing interventions. *Clin. Infect. Dis.* 60 (5): 764–772.

Nelson, D.L. and Cox, M.M. (2015). *Lehninger Principles of Biochemistry.* New York: WH Freeman.

Nshimyiryo, A., Hedt-Gauthier, B., Mutaganzwa, C. et al. (2019). Risk factors for stunting among children under five years: A cross-sectional population-based study in Rwanda using the 2015 Demographic and Health Survey. *BMC Public Health* 19: 175. https://doi.org/10.1186/s12889-019- 6504-z.

Oldenburg, C.E., Guerin, P.J., Berthe, F. et al. (2018). Malaria and nutritional status among children with severe acute malnutrition in Niger: a prospective cohort study. *Clin. Infect. Dis.* 67 (7): 1027–1034.

Pandya, H., Slemming, W., and Saloojee, H. (2018). Health system factors affecting the implementation of integrated management of childhood illness (IMCI): Qualitative insights from a South African province. *Health Policy Plan.* 33 (2): 171–182.

Pribram, V. (2011). *Nutrition and HIV.* United Kingdom: Wiley Blackwell.

Ram, M., Gupte, N., Nayak, U. et al. (2012). Growth patterns among HIV-exposed infants receiving nevirapine prophylaxis in Pune, India. *BMC Infect. Dis.* 12: 282.

Redig, A.J. and Berliner, N. (2013). Pathogenesis and clinical implications of HIV-related anemia in 2013. *Hematol. Am. Soc. Hematol. Educ. Program.* 1: 337–381.

Ruan, S., Wang, W., and Levin, S.A. (2006). The effect of global travel on the spread of SARS. *Math. Biosci. Eng.* 3 (1): 205–218.

Ruel, M.T. and Alderman, H. (2013). Nutrition-sensitive interventions and programmes: how can they help to accelerate progress in improving maternal and child nutrition? *Lancet* 382 (9891): 536–551.

Schaible, U.E. and Kaufmann, S.H.E. (2007). Malnutrition and infection: complex mechanisms and global impacts. *PLoS Med.* 4 (5): e115. https://doi.org/10.1371/journal.pmed.0040115.

Sclar, G.D., Garn, J.V., Penakulapati, G. et al. (2017). Effect of sanitation on cognitive development and school absence: a systematic review. *Int. J. Hyg. Environ. Health* 220 (6): 917–927.

Seddon, J.A. and Shingadia, D. (2014). Epidemiology and Disease Burden of Tuberculosis in Children: A Global Perspective. *Infect. Drug. Resist.* 7: 153–165.

Sharma, M. and Atri, A. (2010). *Essentials of International Health.* Massachusetts: Jones and Bartlett.

Smith, I. (2003). Mycobacterium tuberculosis pathogenesis and molecular determinants of virulence. *Clin. Microbiol. Rev.* 16 (3): 463–496.

Snider, D.E. (1980). Pyridoxine supplementation during isoniazid therapy. *Tubercle* 61 (4): 191–196.

Solomon, F.B., Angore, B.N., Koyra, H.C. et al. (2018). Spectrum of opportunistic infections and associated factors among people living with HIV/AIDS in the era of highly active anti-retroviral treatment in Dawro Zone hospital: a retrospective study. *BMC Res. Notes* 11: 604.

Statistics South Africa (2014). *Mortality and causes of death in South Africa, 2011: Findings from death notification.* Pretoria, Statistics South Africa.

Taguri, A.E., Benimal, I., Mahmud, S.M., and Ahmed, A.M. (2009). Risk factors for stunting among under fives in Libya. *Public Health Nutr.* 12 (8): 1141–1149.

Tate, J.E., Burton, A.H., Boschi-Pinto, C., and Parashar, U.D. (2016). Global, regional, and national estimates of rotavirus mortality in children <5 years of age, 2000-2013. *Clin. Infect. Dis.* 62 (S2): S96–S105.

Taylor-Robinson, D.C., Maavan, N., Donegan, S. et al. (2019). Public health deworming programmes for soil-transmitted helminths in children living in endemic areas. *Cochrane Database Syst. Rev.* 9: CD000371.

Teh, R.N., Sumbele, I.U.N., Meduke, D.N. et al. (2018). Malaria parasitaemia, anaemia and malnutrition in children less than 15 years residing in different altitudes along the slope of Mount Cameroon: prevalence, intensity and risk factors. *Malar. J.* 17 (1): 336.

UNAIDS (2012). *UNAIDS report on the global AIDS pandemic 2012.* Geneva: UNAIDS.

UNICEF, WHO and World Bank (2015). Joint child malnutrition estimates. Global Database on Child Growth and Malnutrition. http://www.who.int/nutgrowthdb/estimates2014/en (accessed January 2019).

United Nations Children's Fund (1997). UNICEF Conceptual Framework. https://www.unicef.org/nutrition/training/2.5/4.html

Vasudevan, A., Lubel, J.S. (2015). New-onset of celiac disease during interferon-based therapy for hepatitis C. *Gastroenterol. Rep.* 3(1): 83–85.

Wallace, A.S., Ryman, T.K., and Dietz, V. (2012). Experiences integrating delivery of maternal and child health services with children immunization programs: Systematic review update. *J. Infect. Dis.* 205 (S1): S6–S19.

Wertheim, J.O. and Worobey, M. (2009). Dating the age of the siv lineages that gave rise to HIV-1 and HIV-2. *PLoS Comput. Biol.* 5 (5): e1000377.

Wheeler, D.A., Gilbert, C.L., Launer, C.A. et al. (1998). Weight loss as a predictor of survival and disease progression in HIV infection. *J. Acquir. Immune Defic. Syndr. Hum. Retrovirol.* 18: 80–85.

Whiteside, A. (2016). *HIV and AIDS: A very short introduction*, 2e. Oxford: Oxford University Press.

WHO (2000). Severe falciparum malaria. World Health Organization communicable diseases cluster. *Trans. R. Soc. Trop. Med. Hyg.* 94 (S1): S1–S9.

WHO (2017). Guidelines for drinking-water quality: fourth edition incorporating the first addendum. Geneva: World Health Organization. Licence: CC BY-NC-SA 3.0 IGO

WHO (2019). *Global Tuberculosis Report 2019.* Geneva: World Health Organisation.

5 Maternal and Child Nutrition

5.1 Introduction

This chapter addresses nutrition during pre-conception and pregnancy, and outlines good infant feeding practices during the first 6 months of life including breastfeeding, complementary feeding from 6 months of age and child nutrition from 12 months of age. It introduces the Innocenti Declaration, highlighting global challenges in meeting targets for maternal and child nutrition, and provides a description of strategies to improve infant and young child feeding practices.

5.2 Nutrition During Pregnancy

Addressing poor nutritional status amongst women of childbearing age is one of the most crucial areas for intervention in improving global health. Evidence from the Dutch famine and the Chinese famine shows that nutrition before and during pregnancy has long-term implications for a chronic disease risk later in life. Maternal overweight and obesity have an impact on birth complications. Micronutrient deficiency in pregnancy can cause problems in foetal growth and development. Nutrients of interest include folate, iron and calcium.

Energy balance is important in supporting the reproductive system. Negative energy balance, where energy expenditure is higher than intake, can result in maternal malnutrition. This results in reduced tissue reserves of nutrients, reduces the ability to conceive and, importantly, increases the risk of preterm birth and intra-uterine growth restriction (IUGR). Preterm birth infants are born before 37 weeks' gestational age. The rate of stillborn infants fell dramatically in England towards the end of the second world war, from 38/1000 births to 28/1000 births, as a result of prioritising food rationing for pregnant and lactating women

Nutrition and Global Health, First Edition. Shawn W. McLaren.
© 2023 John Wiley & Sons Ltd. Published 2023 by John Wiley & Sons Ltd.

(Hytten 1979). A major determinant of IUGR is maternal undernutrition, but other factors include maternal anaemia and infectious diseases including malaria and smoking. IUGR causes infants to be born with a low birthweight (LBW). Both infant birthweight and maternal weight gain are associated with the risk of complications for mother and baby (WHO 1995). A birthweight between 3.1 and 3.6 kg is associated with the optimal ratio of infant and maternal outcomes (WHO 1995). An LBW baby is born from a full-term pregnancy, more than 37 weeks' gestational age, but has a birthweight of less than 2500 g. In addition to the factors associated with IUGR, LBW is also associated with low pre-pregnancy BMI, short maternal stature, poor gestational weight gain, anaemia, infections, smoking and excessive alcohol intake during pregnancy. There is a higher risk of morbidity and mortality for both preterm and LBW infants (Figure 5.1). Both preterm and LBW are associated with reduced cognitive and physical development. There is also an increased risk of chronic diseases in adulthood amongst infants born preterm or with LBW (Barker 1998; Neggers and Goldenberg 2003).

Overweight and obesity are also associated with undesirable reproductive outcomes, including irregular ovulation, higher rates of miscarriage and poly-cystic ovarian syndrome (PCOS). Maternal overweight and obesity are also associated with an increased risk of prolonged labour and are

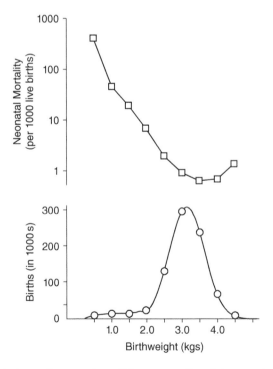

Figure 5.1: The J-shaped curve describing mortality risk associated with different birthweight outcomes (Wilcox 2001).

associated with higher rates of perinatal mortality. Perinatal mortality is defined as the number of stillbirths and deaths that occur in the first week of life per 1000 total births (Villamor and Cnattingius 2006).

Evidence suggests that epigenetic changes occur during gestation amongst infants born to overweight and obese mothers programme individuals for higher risks of overweight, obesity and related non-communicable diseases later in life. These effects are explored in more detail in the chapter on The Nutritional Double Burden of Disease.

However, some countries do not offer official guidelines on weight gain during pregnancy. Most women gain occurs between 10 and 12.5 kg during gestation, the majority of which is gained after week 20. This increase in weight is made up of the baby, the placenta, increased blood volume and adipose tissue, which supports breastfeeding later. It is advised that women do not attempt to lose weight while pregnant, nor should they gain too much weight. Lower weight gains are usually adequate amongst well-nourished women.

5.2.1 Conception

Cell differentiation is rapid immediately after conception. This is a critical time for the developing foetus, and at this stage the pregnancy may be undetected.

The maternal body undergoes physiological changes during pregnancy which affect nutrient availability and turnover. The absorption of nutrients including iron and calcium is increased, and there is an increase in calcium turnover.

Neural tube defects are a concern during pregnancy. While the cause is unknown, it has been established that the maternal diet plays a role and that folic acid supplementation prevents approximately 50% of neural tube defects from occurring. Neural tube defects present as anencephaly, where the foetal brain is absent or fails to develop, encephalocele, which is a protrusion of the brain, and spina bifida, which refers to the incomplete closure of the spinal cord, resulting in a protrusion, as well as damage to nerves and muscles. This may be leg paralysis, loss of sensation or incontinence.

Low intakes of folate are associated with neural tube defects, and women are advised to take folic acid supplements if they are planning to fall pregnant. The recommended dose is 400 ug per day before conception and during the first trimester.

Vitamin A can be teratogenic in very high doses of greater than 3300 µg per day. It is advised that women avoid vitamin A supplements and liver and liver products during pregnancy.

There is no increase in requirements for iron during pregnancy; however, supplementation is common. Iron supplements may be beneficial for women who enter pregnancy with a poor iron status. This is because the iron stores are used to fulfil iron requirements during pregnancy. If iron stores are low at the beginning of pregnancy, the requirements will need to be met through dietary iron (Fernandez-Ballart 2000). Iron supplements may be beneficial for women who enter pregnancy with a poor iron status. While there is an increased physiological demand for iron and calcium during gestation, physiological changes occur which increase the bioavailability of these nutrients from food. Maternal calcium absorption increases from 20 to 30% of calcium ingested at week 24 to approximately 50% in week 36. Maternal iron absorption increases from approximately 7.4% in week 16 to 25.7% in week 36. It should be noted that the increased blood volume in pregnancy results in dilutional anaemia – there is an increase in plasma volume but not in red blood cell count. Plasma volume increases by 45–55%, while red cell volume increases by 18–25% (Broek 2003). This lowers haemoglobin concentration and blood viscosity, which has the effect of improving placental perfusion. Mild anaemia during pregnancy is diagnosed when haemoglobin is between 10.0 and 10.9 g/dl, moderate anaemia in pregnancy is defined as haemoglobin between 7 and 9.9 g/dl and severe anaemia in pregnancy occurs when haemoglobin concentrations fall below 7 g/dl (Broek 2003). All women should be screened for anaemia at least once during pregnancy, and iron supplements should be prescribed if haemoglobin concentrations are below 11 g/dl. Young mothers and teenagers who fall pregnant are at a particularly high risk of anaemia. In addition, multiple pregnancies with close birth spacing, following a vegetarian diet, and hyperemesis gravidarum are factors that can increase the likelihood of anaemia during pregnancy.

There is an increased requirement for calcium during gestation. Retention of calcium in the body increases during pregnancy. Maternal calcium absorption increases from 20 to 30% of calcium ingested at week 24 to approximately 50% in week 36. In addition, the calcium pool in the body increases by approximately 20% over the course of gestation, with calcium turnover rates doubling (Heaney and Skillman 1971). Interestingly, these changes in calcium metabolism begin before most of the calcium deposition takes place in the foetus. It is thought that changes to calcium metabolism are the result of interaction between placental lactogen, oestrogen and parathyroid hormone (Heaney and Skillman 1971).

The WHO has published recommendations on antenatal care (ANC) for a positive pregnancy experience for use within the context of routine ANC across the world. Amongst these recommendations are suggestions for dietary advice and micronutrient supplementation.

In all contexts, pregnant women should be given advice on healthy eating and physical activity during gestation. This is important as excess weight gain during pregnancy can result in negative outcomes for both mother and foetus. In specific contexts where there is a high prevalence of under-nutrition amongst women of childbearing age, the WHO recommends providing nutrition education on protein and energy to prevent LBW infants. In addition, balanced protein and energy supplements are recommended in these populations to prevent small gestational age infants and reduce the risk of stillbirth. However, high protein supplements are not recommended in these populations in pregnancy.

It is recommended that all women take a daily supplement of iron and folic acid in order to prevent complications associated with deficiencies of these nutrients. These complications include anaemia, puerperal sepsis, LBW and stillbirth. Supplementing with 30–60 mg of iron and 0.4 mg folic acid orally per day is recommended. If side effects of supplementation are intolerable or there is a high prevalence of anaemia amongst pregnant women, a weekly oral dose of 120 mg iron and 2.8 mg folic acid may be used instead.

Calcium supplements can be used in populations where calcium intake is low in order to prevent pre-eclampsia. An oral supplement of 1.5–2.0 g per day is appropriate in these populations.

It is recommended that vitamin A supplementation is only given in situations where vitamin A deficiency is a severe public health concern. Vitamin A should be given at a level necessary to prevent night blindness. It should be noted that high doses of vitamin A during gestation can be teratogenic.

5.3 Infant Feeding 0–6 Months

Infants younger than six months old need only breastmilk to grow and thrive. This section discusses the composition of human breastmilk, the benefits of breastfeeding and risks of not breastfeeding.

Birthweight appears to play an important role in neonatal morbidity and mortality risk, as well as having implications for chronic disease risk throughout the life cycle. The rate of weight gain and body composition during the first months of life similarly appear to have implications for health throughout the life cycle. The infant growth trajectory and body composition are closely associated with feeding choices.

Increased relative rates of weight gain during early infancy have been associated with greater fat mass and central adiposity later in life (Chomtho et al. 2008). Therefore, early infancy is a vitally important window of opportunity for managing later chronic disease and obesity risk (Chomtho et al. 2008).

Infants who are fed a breastmilk substitute (formula) have a higher absolute (kg) fat-free mass than breastfed infants throughout the first year of life. Formula-fed infants also have a lower relative (%) fat mass through most of the first year of life compared with breastfed infants, although it appears that relative fat mass is higher amongst formula-fed infants at one year of age (Gale et al. 2012). It is possible that these differences between formula-fed and breastfed infants are due to the fact that total energy expenditure is higher amongst formula-fed infants. It should also be noted that fat-free mass is not made up of skeletal muscle only but also includes bone, organs and smooth muscle tissue. Breastmilk contains leptin that may influence the way that a breastfed infant lays down tissue. In addition, the higher level of adipose tissue deposition observed in breastmilk-fed infants may be a natural adaptation that prepares the infant for the more precarious period of weaning (Gale et al. 2012). In addition to differences in body composition between the formula- and breastfed infant, there are differences in body morphology. The breastfed infant tends to be lighter and taller than the formula-fed infant, which is evident from differences between growth references developed from predominantly formula-fed populations and growth standard references developed from exclusively breastfed populations.

5.3.1 Breastfeeding

- Important aspect of the first 1000 days of life
- Involves hormones oxytocin and prolactin
- Implications for health throughout the life cycle

Breastmilk is produced in the alveoli within the breast tissue (Figure 5.2). It must travel down the lactiferous ducts to exit through the nipple to enter the infant's mouth. The shape or size of the breast does not affect breastmilk supply as this is largely comprised of supporting tissue and fat which does not affect the physiological production of breastmilk. The areola is the region of skin surrounding the nipple. Ensuring a good latch in which some of the areola is in the infant's mouth helps to facilitate feeding and prevent pain and discomfort during feeding. It is recommended that mothers support the breast by cupping the breast above the hand while the infant is latching on instead of exposing the nipple with a 'scissor' configuration (nipple appearing between the index and middle finger) as this second configuration may block the flow of milk through the lactiferous ducts.

Cells secrete breastmilk in the alveoli in response to feeding, which is known as the let down reflex. This mechanism is hormonally regulated. Oxytocin is released in response to suckling, which causes the alveoli to contract, releasing milk. In addition, prolactin is released in response to emptying alveoli, which signals to the alveoli to produce more milk. It is for this reason that infants should be fed regularly (on demand) or to express milk regularly by hand or using a pump, and from both breasts in alteration, in order to maintain milk supply.

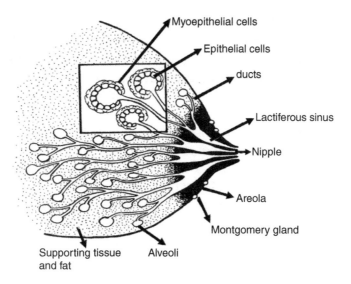

Figure 5.2: Breastfeeding anatomy.

Human breastmilk is all that an infant needs during the first six months in order to survive and thrive. It contains easily digestible proteins as well as enough fluid to keep the infant hydrated. Breastmilk is a dynamic food, and the composition of breastmilk changes in order to meet the infants' needs. Therefore, infants do not need additional water in hot weather if they are breastfeeding. Breastmilk contains additional biological compounds that are not available elsewhere, which support the infant's immune system and give anti-infective properties to the milk. Breastmilk also contains complex carbohydrates that feed the infants gut bacteria, an important quality of breastmilk that has potential implications throughout the life cycle. Amongst the bioactive compounds that have been identified in breastmilk, immune function and antimicrobial activity are supported by the presence of lactoferrin, secretory IgA, osteopontin, cytokines, lysozyme, k-casein, and lacto-peroxidase amongst others (Haschke et al. 2016). Digestive function is supported by bile salt-stimulated lipase, amylase and a1-antitripsin. Growth factors and lactoferrin assist with gut development (Haschke et al. 2016).

Breastfeeding is important for growth, development and health. Poor infant and young child feeding practices are a significant contributor to under-child mortality.

There are short- and long-term benefits to breastfeeding. Breastfeeding lowers the risk of mortality. It lowers the risk of diarrhoea and pneumonia amongst infants (Ip et al. 2009; Lamberti et al. 2011). Breastfeeding lowers the risk of otitis media, an infection of the middle ear which occurs in infants. Therefore, breastfeeding is a protective factor against childhood morbidity and mortality in high-risk regions. The benefits are also seen in high-income populations, where breastfeeding is protective against necrotising enterocolitis and sudden infant death syndrome (Victora et al. 2016). There is evidence that breastfed infants display higher intelligence later in childhood and adulthood (Horta and Victora 2013). Breastfeeding has also been associated with a lower risk of childhood obesity.

The benefits of exclusive breastfeeding are not limited to the infant – there are benefits for the mother as well. These include a reduced risk of post-partum haemorrhage and lower risks of ovarian and breast cancer. It is estimated that current rates of breastfeeding prevent approximately 20 000 deaths from breast cancer annually (Victora et al. 2016). Breastfeeding is a 'natural contraceptive', delaying the return to fertility. It promotes the bond between mother and child.

Preterm infant feeding poses additional challenges. When choosing feeds for preterm infants, the mothers' own breastmilk is the best option. This feeding choice helps to promote the bond between mother and infant, and helps to establish milk supply. If this is unavailable, then donated fresh preterm milk or fresh donated full-term milk is acceptable. Preterm formula is available; however, while the nutrients present are in the correct amounts and proportions, they are less easily digested and lack the biologically active compounds available in breastmilk which support development and immune function. Formula designed for full-term infants is not appropriate for feeding preterm infants as they have different nutrient requirements. This formula is not easily digested by the preterm infant, and its use leads to less than optimum growth and development (Arnold 2006).

5.4 Infant Feeding 6–12 Months

This section discusses the introduction of complementary foods after six months of age.

Complementary feeding refers to introducing foods other than breastmilk to an infant's diet and usually takes place at around six months of age. As breastmilk provides all of the nutrients and fluids that a growing infant need, there is no need to introduce complementary foods before the age of six months. Evidence suggests that early introduction of complementary foods can negatively affect an infant's growth and development, risk of later overweight and obesity (Przyrembel 2012). Breastfeeding appears to protect infants from infection, and early cessation of breastfeeding increases the risk for infections (Przyrembel 2012). It is recommended that weaning is delayed to the age of six months to allow the infants swallow reflex to develop to an appropriate level and for the gut to mature sufficiently to digest foods other than breastmilk.

The WHO recommendations for complementary feeding include the provision that breastfeeding should continue until two years or beyond. It recommends that complementary feeding should involve feeding slowly and patiently, encouraging the infant and talking to the child and making eye contact throughout. Infants should be fed directly, and older children can be assisted with feeding. Parents and caregivers are encouraged to start with small amounts of food and gradually increase the volume, as well as the variety of foods offered. As a guide, infants between six and eight months of age should be given complementary foods two to three times a day, increasing this to three to four meals a day between the ages of nine months and one year. Additional snacks may be included as needed. During times of illness, additional fluids can be given, which may be additional breastfeeds.

There is a current trend towards 'baby-led weaning'. Baby-led weaning refers to the practice of letting infants feed themselves without assistance, allowing them to choose their own foods and does not necessitate pureed, soft or lumpy foods but encourages a variety of textures from the beginning of introducing complementary foods (Pearce and Langely-Evans 2021). Findings from the United Kingdom suggest that baby-led weaning infants are more likely to be breastfed than traditional weaning infants. However, intakes of important nutrients including iron, zinc, iodine, vitamin B12 and vitamin D were significantly higher amongst infants traditionally weaned. In addition, the total energy intake from fat and saturated fat was lower amongst traditionally weaned infants. These differences appear to disappear by nine months of age. Interestingly, a large proportion of caregivers who self-reported baby-led weaning were following practices more objectively similar to traditional weaning practices, suggesting that baby-led weaning is not consistently under-stood or that this practice is socially desirable in this context (Pearce and Langely-Evans 2021).

The first complementary foods introduced should be smooth purees. Home foods including rice, fruit, soft, well-cooked meat, fish, peas, beans and lentils, vegetables and cereals can be offered to infants from six months of age. Eggs and meat should be thoroughly cooked. Complementary foods should be offered before milk feed. Initially, the infant will only eat very small amounts of complementary foods, with the majority of nutritional needs being met by breastmilk (Crawley and Hawdon 2011).

5.4.1 Complementary Feeding Practices

Common indicators of infant and young child feeding practices include tracking early initiation of breastfeeding, exclusive breastfeeding rates, and the proportion of infants and young children meeting minimum dietary diversity and minimum meal frequency. Indicators are outlined in Table 5.1.

Table 5.1: Indicators of infant and young child feeding practices.

Indicator	Meaning	Calculation	Notes
Early initiation of breastfeeding	Proportion of children born in the last 24 months who were put to the breast within 1 hour of birth	Children born in the last 24 months who were put to the breast within 1 hour of birth/children born in the last 24 months	
Exclusive breastfeeding under 6 months	Proportion of infants 0–5 months of age who are fed exclusively with breastmilk	Infants 0–5 months of age who received only breastmilk during the previous day/infants 0–5 months of age	
Exclusive breastfeeding 4–5 months	Proportion of infants 4–5 months of age who are fed exclusively with breastmilk	Infants 4–5 months of age who received only breastmilk during the previous day/infants 4–5 months of age	
Continued breastfeeding at 1 year	Proportion of children 12–15 months of age who are fed breastmilk	Children 12–15 months of age who received breastmilk during the previous day/children 12–15 months of age	
Introduction of solid, semi-solid or soft foods	Proportion of infants 6–8 months of age who receive solid, semi-solid or soft foods	Infants 6–8 months of age who received solid, semi-solid or soft foods during the previous day/infants 6–8 months of age	
Minimum dietary diversity	Proportion of children 6–23 months of age who receive foods from four or more food groups	Children 6–23 months of age who received foods from ≥4 food groups during the previous day/children 6–23 months of age	The sample universe for this indicator is last born children 6–23 months of age living with their mothers. ■ The seven foods groups used for calculation of this indicator are:

(continued)

		■ grains, roots and tubers ■ legumes and nuts ■ dairy products (milk, yogurt and cheese) ■ flesh foods (meat, fish, poultry and liver/organ meats) ■ eggs ■ vitamin-A rich fruits and vegetables ■ other fruits and vegetables.
Minimum meal frequency	Proportion of breastfed and non-breastfed children 6–23 months of age, who receive solid, semi-solid, or soft foods (but also including milk feeds for non-breastfed children) the minimum number of times or more.	Breastfed children 6–23 months of age who received solid, semi-solid or soft foods the minimum number of times or more during the previous day/breastfed children 6–23 months of age and non-breastfed children 6–23 months of age who received solid, semi-solid or soft foods or milk feeds the minimum number of times or more during the previous day/non-breastfed children 6–23 months of age	The sample universe for this indicator is last born children 6–23 months of age living with their mothers. ■ For breastfed children, minimum is defined as 2 times for infants 6–8 months and 3 times for children 9–23 months. For non-breastfed children, minimum is defined as 4 times for children 6–23 months.
Minimum acceptable diet	Proportion of children 6–23 months of age who receive a minimum acceptable diet (apart from breastmilk)	Breastfed children 6–23 months of age who had at least the minimum dietary diversity and the minimum meal frequency during the previous day/breastfed children 6–23 months of age and non-breastfed children 6–23 months of age who received at least two milk feedings and had at least the minimum dietary diversity not including milk feeds and the minimum meal frequency during the previous day/non-breastfed children 6–23 months of age	

Source: Adapted from WHO, USAID, FANTA, AED, UC, DAVIS and IFPI 2008.

Common problems with complementary feeding across the world include poor dietary diversity and meeting the minimum acceptable diet (Ogbo et al. 2015; Na et al. 2018). In Nigeria, there was an improvement in the minimum meal frequency between 2003 and 2013, while the proportion of children receiving the minimum acceptable diet worsened over this time period (Ogbo et al. 2015).

Factors associated with complementary feeding practices include the mothers' education level, socio-economic status and the number of contacts with health services. Minimum dietary diversity is better amongst children with more educated mothers, higher numbers of contacts at health services and higher socio-economic groups (Ogbo et al. 2015). Amongst children in Pakistan, there is poor introduction of complementary foods; however, there have been modest improvements in early child feeding indicators (Hanif 2011). Dietary diversity declined in Bangladesh between 2007 and 2014, with the biggest declines in vitamin A-rich fruits and vegetables (Na et al. 2018). Poor parental education level and low socio-economic status predicted poor complementary feeding practices in this population (Na et al. 2018). Amongst children in Brazil, overall dietary diversity declined between 1998 and 2008; however, there was an increase in fruit consumption (De Oliveira et al. 2014). These findings underline the importance of careful targeting of nutrition interventions to address poor infant and young child feeding practices.

Important factors to consider for appropriate complementary feeding are as follows:

- Viscosity of food
  The viscosity of complementary foods is important. Thin, watery porridges will not have sufficient energy density to support growth. Complementary foods should be viscous enough to stay on a spoon.
- Frequency and duration of feeding
  The frequency and duration of feeding is an important consideration for successful complementary feeding. Breastfeeding on demand, for enough time for an infant or young child to receive both the nutrient dense foremilk and hydrating hind milk, and an appropriate frequency of offering complementary foods will help to ensure that the child receives adequate nutrition for growth and development.
- Nutrient density
  Complementary foods should be nutrient dense foods. After six months of age, body stores of nutrients such as vitamin A and iron will begin to be depleted if they are not replaced through the diet. From six months, breastmilk alone will be insufficient to meet the body's demands for growth. Appropriate nutrient dense foods

include green leafy vegetables, orange and yellow vegetables, and fruits and animal foods such as egg and liver.

- Avoidance of inhibitors and uptake of enhancers

  Micronutrient bioavailability can be inhibited or enhanced by compounds found in commonly consumed foods. Calcium absorption is inhibited by phytic acid. Non-haem iron forms a complex with proteins in beans, reducing its bioavailability. Non-haem iron bioavailability is improved in the presence of vitamin C. Avoiding giving infants and young children tea or coffee can reduce the risk of interference with micronutrient absorption.

- Hygiene, preparation, processing and storage

  In addition, foods need to be culturally acceptable and have a reliable supply and distribution system. Traditionally, it has been recommended that parents and caregivers avoid common allergen foods in the first year of life in order to reduce the risk of allergy development. However, this advice has recently been overturned. The Scientific Advisory Committee on Nutrition (SACN) from the United Kingdom now recommends that cow's milk, eggs, foods containing gluten such as wheat, barley and rye, crushed or pureed nuts and seeds, soy, fish and well-cooked shellfish can be introduced safely from the age of six months.

Anaphylaxis is an important concern for food allergy. However, there are other signs of allergy that should be identified when introducing complementary foods. These include diarrhoea and vomiting, cough, wheezing and shortness of breath, itching and developing rashes, swollen lips, running nose and red eyes. Introducing new complementary foods one at a time and observing for signs of allergy can help to determine whether an allergy has developed.

5.5 Infant Feeding 12 Months and Beyond

This section discusses feeding young children, including nutrition requirements.

After the age of 12 months, children experience a slower rate of growth, but are more physically active. Young children have low nutrient stores and small stomachs. Therefore, nutrient-dense foods are important during this life stage. It is recommended that breastfeeding continues for two years and beyond. The proportion of energy and nutrients provided by breastmilk will reduce as the child consumes more family foods. Approximately 30% of total caloric requirements are still met with breastmilk in the second year of life (WHO 1993). The proportion of total calories provided by fat is higher in this age group as the increased energy density supports growth and brain development. A bulky diet too dilute in nutrients does not provide adequate nutrition for growth. It is important that the diet is not too high in fibre; however, a very low fibre intake can result in constipation in this age group.

Important micronutrients include zinc, calcium, vitamin D and vitamin A. Country-specific healthy eating guidelines are generally introduced from two years of age.

5.6 Initiatives to Promote Exclusive Breastfeeding

Breastmilk banks, the Innocenti Declaration, Kangaroo Mother Care (KMC), the Mother Baby Friendly Initiative (BFI) and the UNICEF 10 Steps to successful breastfeeding are discussed.

The WHO recommendations for breastfeeding success include initiation of breastfeeding within the first hour of life. Early initiation of breastfeeding helps to stimulate milk supply, and the first milk, colostrum, is important for developing the infant's immune system. The WHO recommends exclusive breastfeeding during the first six months of life. This means that infants should receive nothing but breastmilk for the first six months of life, and no additional foods or drinks, including water, should be introduced. Breastmilk contains all the nutrients and fluid that the infant requires and adapts to the infant's needs. Breastfeeding should be on demand, as often as the infant wants to feed, day or night. The WHO also recommends avoiding the use of bottles, teats and pacifiers as this can result in nipple confusion and reduce breastfeeding success.

Strategies to promote exclusive breastfeeding include public health campaigns to promote EBF and discussing infant feeding strategies as early as possible in antenatal clinic visits. Advice from health workers should include a discussion of the benefits and risks of infant feeding strategies. The partner should be included if possible, as this promotes support for the mother.

The WHO has developed the 10 Steps to successful breastfeeding to ensure that health facilities are supportive of breastfeeding. Adopting the WHO 10 Steps helps to ensure that all staff, both clinical and non-clinical, in healthcare settings, are aware of their roles in promoting exclusive breastfeeding.

WHO 10 steps to successful breastfeeding:

1. Have a written breastfeeding policy that is routinely communicated to all healthcare staff.
2. Train all healthcare staff in skills necessary to implement this policy.

3. Inform all pregnant women about the benefits and management of breastfeeding.
4. Help mothers initiate skin-to-skin contact and breastfeeding within a half-hour of birth.
5. Show mothers how to breastfeed and how to maintain lactation even if they should be separated from their infants.
6. Give newborn infants no food or drink other than breastmilk unless medically indicated.
7. Practice rooming-in allows mothers and infants to remain together 24 hours a day.
8. Encourage breastfeeding on demand.
9. Give no artificial teats or pacifiers (also called dummies or soothers) to breastfeeding infants
10. Foster the establishment of breastfeeding support groups and refer mothers to them upon discharge from the hospital or clinic.

Perinatal strategies to promote EBD include assisting the mother to make an informed decision on her infant feeding strategy prior to delivery. Supporting normal vaginal delivery (NVD) births helps to prevent delays to early initiation in breastfeeding.

The mother BFI is an important campaign to create environments supportive of breastfeeding. The Mother BFI was launched by UNICEF in 1991. The aims of the initiative were to support the implementation of the WHO 10 Steps to successful breastfeeding in hospitals and maternity facilities. This has since been expanded to universities offering midwifery and nursing courses. Facilities that are compliant with the 10 Steps are accredited by UNICEF.

5.6.1 Kangaroo Mother Care

Neonatal ICU is a challenging environment for breastfeeding. Emotional distress around the time of delivery and discharge from hospital may be present although these tend to subside over time (Callen et al. 2005). Low milk volume is a barrier to breastfeeding amongst mothers of infants in the NICU (Callen et al. 2005). Nipple and breast problems are also common barriers in NICU settings (Callen et al. 2005). Following discharge from the NICU, a poor breastfeeding technique is a problem a month after discharge, and between one and three months after discharge the weak physical status of premature infants makes breastfeeding challenging (Callen et al. 2005).

Emotional distress has a negative effect on milk supply as oxytocin and prolactin are affected. Conventional neonatal care for premature and LBW infants also means that there is a large amount of separation between mother and infant, which can interfere with sustained milk supply.

KMC has been introduced as an alternative to conventional neonatal care for low birthweight infants. KMC began as a general post-delivery strategy, encouraging skin-to-skin contact, frequent and exclusive breast-feeds and avoidance of late discharge from the hospital following delivery. Applying KMC principles to LBW and premature infants has been shown to reduce the mortality risk of infants, as well as the risk of nosocomial infection and hypothermia (Conde-Agudelo and Díaz-Rossello 2016). Therefore, KMC is a valuable alternative neonatal care policy for low birthweight infants in resource-poor settings (Conde-Agudelo and Díaz-Rossello 2016).

Postnatal strategies to promote EBF rely on a solid foundation developed during the antenatal and perinatal stages. Strategies after delivery should aim to promote continued breastfeeding. This may include breast-feeding support groups, provision of individual counselling, growth monitoring and promotion campaigns and optimising the use of routine contacts, such as visits to clinics for routine vaccinations to discuss challenges in maintaining breastfeeding.

Practical strategies for implementing the WHO 10 Steps:

1. **Have a written breastfeeding policy that is routinely communicated to all healthcare staff**

   The breastfeeding policy should be communicated to all new staff. Opportunities for communicating the policy include regularly scheduled in-service training sessions and informal discussions. New staff should receive orientation on the MBFI policy. Staff members should be encouraged to participate in annual reviews of the policy, updating contents and including the latest evidence-based practice.

   A summarised version of the policy including the 10 Steps and support for non-breastfeeding mothers should be displayed in appropriate areas of healthcare facilities. Support for non-breastfeeding mothers could focus on cup feeding. This could be in the form of posters. Good areas to include posters are maternal and obstetrics departments and antenatal departments, but they do not need to be limited to these areas. It may be a good idea to include local language versions of these posters in wording which can easily be understood.

2. **Train all healthcare staff in skills necessary to implement this policy**

   Plan for regular staff training on the breastfeeding policy. In-service training could focus on aspects of the policy and infant and young child feeding-related skills. Ideas for in-service training may include communication skills, practices that assist breastfeeding, promoting breastfeeding during pregnancy, helping with breastfeeding, breast and nipple conditions and complications, maternal health concerns and continued support for breastfeeding mothers. Staff could be encouraged to participate in breastfeeding and lactation management courses.

Staff will also need to be trained on safe breastmilk substitute preparation, storage and cup feeding for infants who are not breast-fed. This training should pay careful attention to the International Code of Marketing Breastmilk Substitutes. Staff members should be trained to discourage bottle feeding in waiting areas and consulting rooms. Instead, mothers of non-breastfed infants should be encouraged to feed their infants with cups. Pacifiers, soothers and dummies should similarly be discouraged in waiting areas. Breastfeeding mothers should be encouraged to breastfeed their infants in any area that is conducive to the practice and should be praised for breastfeeding by passing members of staff.

3. **Inform all pregnant women about the benefits and management of breastfeeding**

Opportunities should be used or created to remind women and their partners about the benefits of breastfeeding. This may be during one-to-one consultations, group talks in waiting areas and informal discussions. The same opportunities can be used to discuss the risks of the early introduction of complementary foods.

4. **Help mothers initiate skin-to-skin contact and breastfeeding within a half-hour of birth**

Policy within maternal and obstetric units (MOU) could include a requirement for babies to receive at least 60 minutes of skin-to-skin contact with their mothers immediately after birth. Mothers should be encouraged to breastfeed immediately after delivery and show how to look for signs that the baby is ready to breastfeed, offering help as needed. KMC should be included in MOU policy to promote wellness and survival amongst premature and low birthweight infants.

5. **Show mothers how to breastfeed and how to maintain lactation even if they should be separated from their infants**

Further help with breastfeeding should be offered to mothers in the hours following delivery. All breastfeeding mothers should be shown how to position the baby correctly for breastfeeding and signs of a good latch. Hand expression of breastmilk should be taught to breastfeeding mothers. Leaflets could be designed as reminders for mothers when they return home and could include details of who to contact for further assistance. Mothers who have opted not to breastfeed should be informed of the risks of not breastfeeding but must be shown how to prepare the feeds they have chosen. Facilities may have dedicated milk kitchens for preparing infant formula or small demonstration kitchens for showing mothers how to safely prepare a breastmilk substitute feed.

6. **Give newborn infants no food or drink other than breast-milk unless medically indicated**

   No water, infant formula or other foods or drinks should be given to infants younger than six months of age unless they are medically indicated or if the parents have made a fully informed choice. It is good practice to document to reason for supplementary feeds or other foods or fluids given in the relevant patient documents.

7. **Practice rooming-in allows mothers and infants to remain together 24 hours a day**

   Rooming-in needs to include both the day and night, and the mother should be encouraged to maintain constant concern for her infant's well-being. The mother and infant should not be separated unjustifiably, and the reasons for separation need to be recorded in the patient documents.

8. **Encourage breastfeeding on demand**

   Teach mothers how to recognise signs that the baby is hungry and when they have finished feeding. Avoid placing restrictions on the frequency and duration of breastfeeding. Encourage mothers to breastfeed their infants whenever they are hungry and in any area of the healthcare facility. Mothers should also be informed that they may wake their infants up, even at night, to breastfeed if the breasts are overfull or uncomfortable.

9. **Give no artificial teats or pacifiers (also called dummies or soothers) to breastfeeding infants**

   Prevent breastfeeding infants from being given bottles or teats, and ensure that mothers are informed of the risks involved in using bottles. Prevent breastfeeding babies from being given pacifiers or dummies.

10. **Foster the establishment of breastfeeding support groups and refer mothers to them upon discharge from the hospital or clinic**

    Provide information on where to access help and support with breastfeeding at home and provide directions and information to the nearest day clinic. Healthcare workers can work with community-based mother support groups and other community services. When mothers and their infants are discharged after delivery, their discharge plan should include follow-up details. The mother should also be given emergency contact details for the health facility.

5.6.2 Updates to the Mother Baby Friendly Initiative—the Baby Friendly Initiative

UNICEF updated the approach of the mother BFI in 2013 and has since then replaced the MBFI with the BFI. The newer BFI is divided into three stages of implementation. Stage 1 is building a firm foundation. Stage 2 is an educated workforce. Stage 3 is parents' experiences.

Stage 1: Building a firm foundation
   The main actions for this initial stage of implementing the BFI include having a written policy and guidelines to support the standards. Institutions are required to have an education plan in place to allow staff to implement the standards according to their role. Institutions will also need to set up processes for implementing, monitoring and evaluating the standards. While building a firm foundation, institutions should ensure that there is no promotion of breastmilk substitutes, bottles, teats or pacifiers in the facility.

Stage 2: An educated workforce
   During this stage, all staff members of the facility which is to be given baby-friendly accreditation should be educated on how they will implement the standards according to their role.

Stage 3: Parents' experiences
   For the final stage of accreditation with the BFI, different types of facilities will need to meet different requirements that are particular to the setting.

In maternity service settings, facilities and their staff must support pregnant women in recognising the importance of breastfeeding and early relationships with their baby. This is to underline the importance of these factors in the health and well-being of the baby. Facilities and staff should support the initiation of breastfeeding soon after birth. They should encourage bonding between mother and baby. Mothers should be supported to get breastfeeding off to a good start. Support should be given to ensure that mothers make informed decisions about starting their infants on foods and fluids other than breastmilk. Parents and their babies should be supported to have a close and loving relationship.
   Neonatal units such as neonatal intensive care present additional challenges for feeding infants and maintain breastfeeding and breastmilk production. Within neonatal units, parents must be supported to have a close and loving relationship with their baby. Infants should receive breastmilk or be encouraged to breastfeed wherever possible. Parents must be valued as partners in the care that the infant receives.

BFI must extend to community nursing services in order to promote and protect continued breastfeeding. In community nursing settings, women should be encouraged to recognise the importance of breastfeeding and early relationships with their infants right from pregnancy. Mothers should be enabled to continue breastfeeding for as long as they wish. Mothers should be supported to make informed decisions on introducing foods and fluids other than breastmilk to their infants.

5.7 Challenges in Infant and Young Child Feeding

There are low breastfeeding rates across the world. This section explores barriers to successful breastfeeding, including support for women, the breastmilk substitute market, and the early introduction of complementary foods.

Barriers to better breastfeeding rates are related to the breastfeeding environment. For successful breastfeeding to take place, a supportive, enabling environment is required. In addition, breastfeeding needs to be a collective societal responsibility and not simply the mother's responsibility only. The breastmilk substitute market is part of the environment surrounding supporting breastfeeding, and advertising, growth and the social aspects of breastmilk substitute use of impacts on breastfeeding rates. Barriers to successful breastfeeding also include unrecognised health and economic costs of not breastfeeding, resulting in poor support of the practice. Successful breastfeeding and improved breastfeeding initiation and continuation require political and financial support and investment (Rollins et al. 2016).

5.7.1 The Innocenti Declaration

The Innocenti Declaration was produced to address some of these barriers to successful breastfeeding. The Innocenti Declaration was adopted at the WHO/UNICEF policymakers' meeting on 'Breastfeeding in the 1990s: A Global Initiative', held at Spedale degli Innocenti, Florence, Italy, in August 1990. The meeting was co-sponsored by USAID and the Swedish International Development Authority (SIDA). The main action points agreed upon in the Innocent Declaration relate to adopting the WHO 10 Steps to successful breastfeeding, the international code for marketing breastmilk substitutes and protecting the rights of breastfeeding women. Within the Innocenti Declaration, member states agree that every facility providing maternity services fully practises all 10 of the 10 Steps to successful breastfeeding. The Declaration gave effect to all articles contained in the International Code of Marketing of Breastmilk Substitutes. Finally, legislation protecting the rights of breastfeeding women and the means for enforcing this legislation were agreed.

5.7.2 International Code of Marketing of Breastmilk Substitutes

The International Code of Marketing of Breastmilk Substitutes was adopted by the World Health Assembly in 1981 and acts as a health policy framework.

Article 5: The general public and mothers

- 5.1 There should be no advertising or other form of promotion to the general public of products within the scope of this code.
- 5.2 Manufacturers and distributors should not provide, directly or indirectly, samples of products within the scope of this code to pregnant women, mothers or members of their families.
- 5.3 In conformity with paragraphs 1 and 2 of this Article, there should be no point-of-sale advertising, giving of samples or any other promotion device to induce sales directly to the consumer at the retail level, such as special displays, discount coupons, premiums, special sales, loss-leaders and tie-in sales, for products within the scope of this code. This provision should not restrict the establishment of pricing policies and practices intended to provide products at lower prices on a long-term basis.
- 5.4 Manufacturers and distributors should not distribute any gifts of articles or utensils to pregnant women or mothers or infants and young children which may promote the use of breastmilk substitutes or bottle feeding.
- 5.5 Marketing personnel, in their business capacity, should not seek direct or indirect contact of any kind with pregnant women or with mothers of infants and young children.

5.7.3 Trends in Breastmilk Substitute Use

The International Code of Marketing of Breastmilk Substitutes aims to reduce the negative effects of sub-optimal breastfeeding globally. However, research has shown that breastmilk substitute sales have increased over the period 2008–2013 (Baker et al. 2016). Sales increased from 5.5 to 7.8 kg of breastmilk substitute per child per year over this period. The fastest growth in sales occurred in East Asia, and increases in sales are associated with increased country income levels (Baker et al. 2016). The increases in breastmilk the breastmilk substitute market are concerning for global child and maternal health, and suggest that more efficacious strategies are required to regulate sales of breastmilk substitutes (Baker et al. 2016).

5.7.3.1 Assessing the Impact of IYCF

Despite strategies to improve infant and young child feeding practices, evidence suggests that childhood anthropometry has not been affected by breastfeeding promotion activities (Giugliani et al. 2015). More intensive strategies to promote good breastfeeding practices have been shown to improve rates of early initiation of breastfeeding and continued exclusive breastfeeding (Menon et al. 2016).

5.8 Conclusion

High-income countries have shorter breastfeeding duration than low- and middle-income countries. However, even in low- and middle-income countries, only 37% of infants younger than six months are exclusively breastfed.

The scaling up of breastfeeding can prevent an estimated 823 000 child deaths and 20 000 breast cancer deaths every year.

Findings from studies conducted with modern biological techniques suggest novel mechanisms that characterise breastmilk as a personalised medicine for infants.

Breastfeeding promotion is important in developed and developing countries alike and might contribute to achievement of the Sustainable Development Goals.

References

Arnold, L. (2006). Global health policies that support the use of banked donor human milk: a human rights issue. *Int. Breastfeeding J.* https://doi.org/10.11 86/1746-4358-1-26.

Baker, P., Smith, J., Salmon, L. et al. (2016). Global trends and patterns of commercial milk-based formula sales: is an unprecedented infant and young child feeding transition underway? *Public Health Nutr.* 20 (1): 165–173.

Broek (2003). *Anaemia and Micronutrient Deficiencies*. British Medical Bulletin.

Callen, J., Pinelli, J., Atkinson, S., and Saigal, S. (2005). Qualitative analysis of barriers to breastfeeding in very-low-birthweight infants in the hospital and postdischarge. *Adv. Neonatal Care* 5 (2): 93–103.

Chomtho, S., Wells, J.C.K., Williams, J.E. et al. (2008). Infant growth and later body composition: evidence from the 4-compartment model. *Am. J. Clin. Nutr.* 87 (6): 1776–1784.

Conde-Agudelo, A. and Díaz-Rossello, J.L. (2016). Kangaroo mother care to reduce morbidity and mortality in low birthweight infants. *Cochrane Database Syst. Rev.* 8: CD002771. https://doi.org/10.1002/14651858.CD002771.pub4.

Crawley, H. and Hawdon, D. (2011). *Eating Well: First Year of Life Practical Guide.* The Caroline Walker Trust.

De Oliveira, D., de Castro, I.R.R., and Jaime, P.C. (2014). Complementary feeding patterns in the first year of life in the city of Rio de Janeiro, Brazil: time trends from 1998 to 2008. *Cad. Saude Publica* 30 (8): 1755–1764.

Fernandez-Ballart, J.D. (2000). Iron metabolism during pregnancy. *Clin. Drug Investig.* 19: 9–19.

Gale, C., Logan, K.M., Santhakumaran, S. et al. (2012). Effect of breastfeeding compared with formula feeding on infant body composition: a systematic review and meta-analysis. *Am. J. Clin. Nutr.* 95 (3): 656–669.

Giugliani, E.R.J., Horta, B.L., de Mola, C.L. et al. (2015). Effect of breastfeeding promotion interventions on child growth: a systematic review and meta-analysis. *Acta Paediatr.* 104 (467): 20–29.

Hanif, H.M. (2011). Trends in breastfeeding and complementary feeding practices in Pakistan, 1990–2007. *Int. Breastfeeding J.* 6: 15.

Haschke, F., Haiden, N., and Thakkar, S.K. (2016). Nutritive and bioactive proteins in breastmilk. *Ann. Nutr. Metab.* 69 (2): 17–26.

Heaney, R.P. and Skillman, T.G. (1971). Calcium metabolism in normal human pregnancy. *J. Clin. Endocrinol. Metab.* 33 (4): 661–670.

Horta, B.L. and Victora, C.G. (2013). *Long-Term Effects of Breastfeeding: A Systematic Review.* Geneva, Switzerland: World Health Organisation.

Hytten (1979). Nutrition in pregnancy. *Postgrad. Med. J.* 55: 295–302.

Ip, S., Chung, M., Raman, G. et al. (2009). A summary of the Agency for Healthcare Research and Quality's evidence report on breastfeeding in developed countries. *Breastfeed. Med.* 4 (1): S17–S30.

Lamberti, L.M., Walker, C.L.F., Noiman, A. et al. (2011). Breastfeeding and the risk of diarrhea morbidity and mortality. *BMC Public Health* 11 (3): S15.

Menon, P., Nguyen, P.H., Saha, K.K. et al. (2016). Impacts on breastfeeding practices of at-scale strategies that combine intensive interpersonal counseling, mass media, and community mobilization: results of cluster-randomized program evaluations in Bangladesh and Viet Nam. *PLoS One* 13 (10): e1002159. https://journals.plos.org/plosmedicine/article?id=10.1371/journal.pmed.100215.

Na, M., Aguayo, V.M., Arimond, M. et al. (2018). Stagnating trends in complementary feeding practices in Bangladesh: an analysis of national surveys from 2004–2014. *Matern. Child Nutr.* 14 (S4): e12624.

Ogbo, F.A., Page, A., Idoko, J. et al. (2015). Trends in complementary feeding indicators in Nigeria, 2003–2013. *Br. Med. J. Open* 5: e008467. https://doi.org/10.1136/bmjopen-2015-008467.

Pearce, J. and Langely-Evans, S.C. (2021). Comparison of food and nutrient intake in infants aged 6–12 months, following baby-led or traditional weaning: a cross-sectional study. *J. Hum. Nutr. Diet.* https://doi.org/10.1111/jhn.12947.

Przyrembel, H. (2012). Timing of introduction of complementary food: short- and long-term health consequences. *Ann. Nutr. Metab.* 60 (S2): 8–20.

Rollins, N.C., Bhandari, N., Hajeebhoy, N. et al. (2016). Why invest? And what will it take to improve breastfeeding practices? *Lancet* 387 (10017): 491–504.

Victora, C.G., Bahl, R., Barros, A.J.D. et al. (2016). Breastfeeding in the 21st century: epidemiology, mechanisms and lifelong effect. *Lancet* 387: 475–490.

Villamor, E. and Cnattingius, S. (2006). Interpregnancy weight change and risk of adverse pregnancy outcomes: a population-based study. *Lancet* 368: 1164–1170.

WHO (1995). *WHO Collaborative Study on Maternal Anthropometry and Pregnancy Outcomes*. Geneva: World Health Organisation.

WHO, USAID, FANTA, AED, UC, DAVIS, IFPI (2008). *Indicators for Assessing Infant and Young Child Feeding Practices*. Geneva, Switzerland: World Health Organisation.

Barker, D.J. (1998). In utero programming of chronic disease. *Clin. Sci. (London)* 95 (2): 115–128.

Neggers, Y. and Goldenberg, R.L. (2003). Some thoughts on body mass index, micronutrient intakes and pregnancy outcome. *J. Nutr.* 133 (5S2): 1737S–1740S.

World Health Organization (1993). Division of Diarrhoeal and Acute Respiratory Disease Control & United Nations Children's Fund (UNICEF). In: *Breastfeeding counselling: a training course*. World Health Organization.

Wilcox, A.J. (2001). On the importance- and the unimportance- of birthweight. *Int. J. Epidemiol.* 30 (6): 1233–1241.

6 Childhood Malnutrition

The effects of inadequate nutrition include linear growth retardation (known as stunting), poor weight gain resulting in underweight and the loss of lean and adipose tissue (also referred to as wasting). While each of these conditions results from some degree of undernutrition, the differences in their aetiologies are explored.

The three main forms of malnutrition amongst children result in poor weight gain, poor linear growth or weight loss. Poor weight gain is called 'underweight', and it means that a child is small for their age. Poor linear growth is referred to as 'stunting', when a child is too short for their age. Wasting occurs when a child has lost weight rapidly and is thin for their attained height. Undernutrition in childhood is associated with a high risk of mortality (Mwangome et al. 2012).It is also associated with poor cognitive development in children (Fink and Rockers 2014). The number of years of education a child receives, and the likelihood of failing a year at school, is significantly associated with weight gain in the first two years of life. Furthermore, catch-up growth amongst children born as low birthweight infants is associated with an increased number of years of education (Maluccio et al. 2009). Good nutritional status in early childhood is an important economic developmental issue.

There is evidence that malnutrition during childhood predisposes people to an increased risk of overweight and obesity (Figure 6.1), as well as the associated chronic diseases of lifestyle in adulthood (Pedro et al. 2014; Prendergast and Humphrey 2014). Stunted children do not meet their height potential, and this results in a shorter stature in adulthood (Haddinott et al. 2013), which raises body mass index (BMI) as BMI weight is high relative to height. The nutritional status of children is therefore an extremely important determinant of their long-term health and is the result of many social, economic and cultural factors (Schoeman et al. 2010).

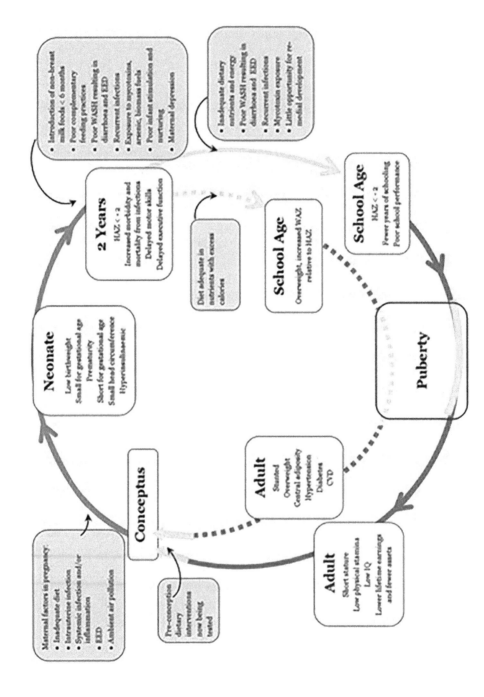

Figure 6.1: Causes and consequences of stunting throughout the life cycle (Prendergast and Humphrey 2014).

6.1 Stunting

The global prevalence of stunting is decreasing (Black et al. 2013). The global prevalence for stunting was 39.3% of children in 1990, equating to approximately 252 million children. The estimated number of stunted children worldwide had reduced to 20.8% of children (141.3 million children) in 2020 and is predicted to decrease further to 17.2% or 116.5 million children by 2030 (WHO 2020). These improvements in stunting prevalence are not spread uniformly across the world, with some regions performing better than others. The African region had a stunting prevalence of 42.2% (46.3 million children) in 1990, which was reduced to 28.7% (57.4 million children) in 2020. While the relative stunting prevalence has decreased by 13.5%, the absolute number of stunted children has actually increased as the population has grown. In Asia, the prevalence of stunting has halved from 47.5% (189.3 million children) in 1990 to 21.2% (75.8 million children) in 2020, representing an improvement of 26.3%. In Central America, the prevalence of stunting has decreased from 31.9% (5.1 million children) in 1990 to 12.1% (1.9 million children) in 2020. Latin America and the Caribbean were predicted to more than halve the prevalence of stunting between 1990 and 2020.

6.2 Causes of Stunting

Stunting as a form of growth deficit was first differentiated from wasting in the 1970s by Waterlow. The introduction of the height for age growth index allowed clinicians, researchers and policymakers to distinguish between low weight attainment due to short stature versus emaciation. This development had important implications for public health policy.

Traditionally, stunting was thought to result from a deficit in macronutrient intakes, and later micronutrient deficiency was thought to play a role in its development in children. Research into the differences in growth trajectory between breastfed and breastmilk substitute fed children led to the theory that early childhood nutrition and breastfeeding and complementary feeding practices were factors that predispose children to a likelihood of stunting. More recently, scholars have begun to identify that stunting has a wide range of risk factors that are broader than infant and young child feeding and include the intrauterine growth environment, birthweight, maternal stature, maternal education level and poverty. The relationship between infection and malnutrition is also an important area in stunting aetiology. Environmental enteric dysfunction resulting in subclinical inflammation in the gut is thought to affect nutrient absorption and utilisation. This links access to clean water and sanitation, soil transmitted helminths and stunting risk.

Keino et al. (2014) linked the increased prevalence of stunting with socioeconomic, demographic and environmental factors amongst children aged less than five years in sub-Saharan Africa. These researchers found that there was a direct link between stunting and the mothers' education, occupation and household income. People residing in rural areas, especially males, were more vulnerable to stunting. Additionally, low birthweight, short maternal stature and history of not taking deworming medication during pregnancy were associated with a higher risk of stunting amongst Rwandan children (Nshimyiryo et al. 2019).

Similar results were observed in India, where Chowdhury et al. (2013) showed that the risk of stunting amongst children between six and 59 months old was significantly related to socio-economic factors. The risk of stunting in children was higher amongst those households with reduced buying power and access to resources because of unemployment (Chowdhury et al. 2013). Stunting was also significantly higher amongst males and in younger infants (Chowdhury et al. 2013).

Amongst the causes of stunting described by the Conceptual Framework on Stunting (Figure 6.2) (Stewart et al. 2013) are poor micronutrient quality, low dietary diversity and intake of animal foods, the anti-nutrient content of the diet and low energy content of complementary foods. In a study of internally-displaced people, Ali et al. (2015) found that there was an association between late and early weaning and undernutrition in children. Complementary feeding was initiated before six months of age in 52% of their sample. A delayed introduction to complementary food was also associated with undernutrition (stunting, wasting and underweight for age) (Ali et al. 2015). Apart from that, a large family size was positively associated with wasting, stunting and underweight for age (Ali et al. 2015). Dietary diversity and the number of meals eaten per day were linked with stunting in a study on Ethiopian children younger than five years old (Motbainor et al. 2015).

Stunting prevalence differed significantly between urban and rural groups of Peruvian children (Pomeroy et al. 2014). According to Pomeroy et al. (2014), rural children appear to be at a higher risk of stunting. Stunting was also significantly associated with the duration of exclusive breastfeeding and choosing to exclusively formula feed in India (Chowdhury et al. 2013).

The risk of stunting in children was associated with having student/ younger mothers (Mamabolo et al. 2005). With a teenage fertility rate of 52 per 1000 adolescent girls for the years 2006–2009 (Makiwane 2010), this could contribute to stunting in South Africa.

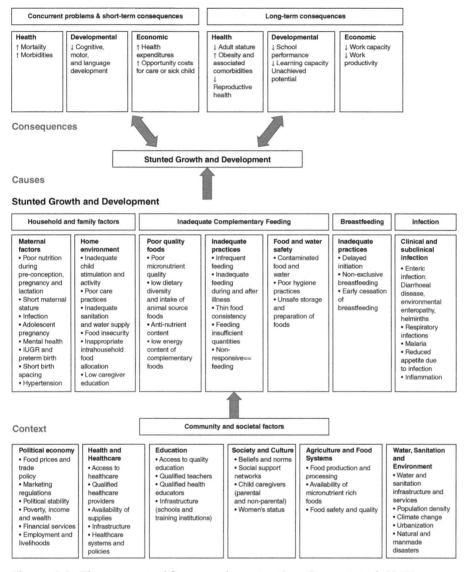

Figure 6.2: The conceptual framework on stunting (Stewart et al. 2013).

6.3 Prevention and Treatment of Stunting

Haddinott et al. (2013) have suggested that investing in strategies that have been proven to reduce stunting amongst children will have extremely favourable economic outcomes in the long term. These strategies include universal salt iodization, multiple micronutrient supplementation, community-based intervention strategies for improving breastfeeding and complementary feeding strategies, and community-based management of severe acute malnutrition (SAM) (Haddinott et al. 2013). Applying the strategies intended to reduce stunting as suggested by Haddinott et al. (2013) results in a benefit:cost ratio of between 3.5 (Democratic Republic of Congo) and 24.4 (Nigeria) in the sub-Saharan African context.

The contribution to stunting reduction is comparable to health and nutrition sectors and other sectors – that is, nutrition-sensitive interventions are approximately as effective at reducing stunting on scale as nutrition-specific interventions as detailed by Haddinott et al. (2013) (Bhutta et al. 2020). According to Bhutta et al. (2020), improvements in maternal education, reductions in fertility or wider birth spacing, and improvements in maternal and newborn care are all interventions that can effectively reduce the prevalence of stunting.

6.3.1 Severe Acute Malnutrition

6.3.1.1 Introduction

Great progress has been made in reducing the number of child deaths globally. The World Health Organisation (WHO) has reported that the under-five mortality rate has reduced by 58% between 1990 and 2017 (World Health Organisation 2017). However, 5.4 million children still died before their fifth birthday during 2017, a rate of 39 per 1000 live births (WHO 2017).

Malnutrition is estimated to contribute to 45% of all under-five child deaths (WHO 2013, 2017). SAM is a common comorbidity amongst children younger than five years admitted to hospitals in developing regions (Gachau et al. 2018). Understanding acute malnutrition, its prevention and treatment is an important step in achieving the Sustainable Development Goal of ending child deaths by 2030.

6.3.1.2 Defining Acute Malnutrition

Acute malnutrition is caused by insufficient dietary intake or illness. SAM is a condition characterised by severe wasting, anorexia, micronutrient deficiency, electrolyte imbalance and oedema and dehydration.

SAM has three broad clinical forms: marasmus, kwashiorkor and marasmic kwashiorkor. In the past, kwashiorkor was attributed to a deficiency of protein and marasmus to energy deficiency. Due to these assumed causes, kwashiorkor and marasmus were collectively termed protein energy malnutrition. However, this thinking was later challenged by research that showed that the diets of children with marasmus and kwashiorkor are not different; therefore, it is unlikely that either manifestation can be attributed to either protein or energy deficit on its own. In addition, physiological homeostasis could not be restored by treatment based on protein energy malnutrition concepts. Therefore, current thinking underpinning the treatment of SAM recognises that the condition is caused by a deficiency of a wide range of nutrients, including potassium, magnesium, phosphate and energy and macronutrients, all of which contribute to poor appetite and wasting.

> *Marasmus and kwashiorkor are common terms historically used to differentiate between types of SAM. Marasmus refers to children who are very thin for their height (that is, they meet the weight-for-height Z-scores (WHZ) or mid-upper arm circumference (MUAC) cut-off) but do not have bilateral pitting oedema; kwashiorkor refers to oedematous malnutrition. The most recent WHO terminology for SAM has replaced these terms.*

6.3.2 Black et al. (2016)

SAM is defined by two distinct clinical entities. Severe wasting or marasmus is defined as a child between birth and 59 months with $WHZ < -3$ Z-scores according to the WHO 2006 growth standards. Kwashiorkor presents with bilateral pitting oedema and is differentiated from marasmus by the presence of nutritional oedema.

The updated terminology divides acute malnutrition into uncomplicated SAM and complicated SAM. Uncomplicated SAM children present without signs of infection are otherwise clinically well, with no other indication for hospital admission. In uncomplicated SAM cases, children pass an appetite test. Retained appetite indicates the absence of severe metabolic disturbance.

Complicated SAM cases present with clinical features of infection, metabolic disturbance, severe oedema, hypothermia, vomiting, severe dehydration, severe anaemia or a lack of appetite. These children require inpatient treatment with low-protein milk based feeds.

6.3.3 Causes of Acute Malnutrition (Figure 6.3)

Direct causes of acute malnutrition include illness and infection (Rahman et al. 2009) and inadequate dietary intake (Steenkamp et al. 2016; Rytter et al. 2015; Rahman et al. 2009). Acute malnutrition is caused by household food insecurity and poor dietary diversity. These issues are prevalent in regions affected by poverty, war and natural disaster. Infectious diseases including HIV, tuberculosis and gastroenteritis are linked to acute malnutrition. Research suggests that there are strong associations between HIV and HFA and WFA in children (Kimani-Murage 2013). Children who experience repeated infections after weaning suffer from mucosal dysfunction, systemic metabolic responses, impaired intake, malabsorption and altered immune responses, which result in malnutrition (Mata 1992).

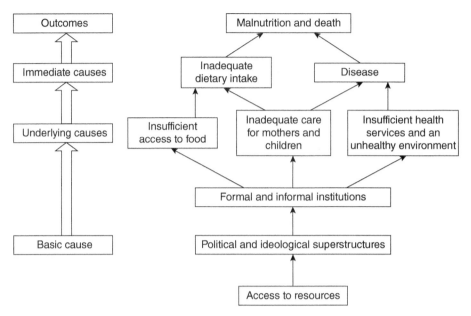

Figure 6.3: UNICEF Conceptual Framework on the Causes of Malnutrition (UNICEF 1990).

6.3.3.1 Screening and Diagnosing Acute Malnutrition

Children are identified in the community by trained community health workers by assessing the weight for height Z-score chart, mid-upper arm circumference and the presence of bilateral pitting oedema (Figure 6.4). Children are then referred to a treatment centre for a full assessment that includes a medical examination and interpretation of the weight-for-height Z-score chart. The treatment algorithms for acute malnutrition depend on the severity of malnutrition, the presence of complications and lack of appetite (Brown et al. 2009).

The WHO recommends using WHZ or weight-for-length (WFL) Z-scores to identify children with SAM (WHO 2013). MUAC is also suggested by the WHO as a diagnostic tool for identifying acute malnutrition in children between six and 60 months of age (WHO 2013). Children with a WHZ below −3 standard deviations (SD) of the WHO standard for children less than 60 months of age have a greatly elevated risk of death compared to children with a WHZ above −3 SD of this standard (WHO 2006). The WHO therefore recommends the use of a WHZ of below −3 SD from the WHO standard to identify children with SAM (WHO 2013; WHO and UNICEF 2009). An MUAC measurement of below 11.5 cm is also recommended to identify SAM in children between six and 60 months of age (WHO 2013; WHO and UNICEF 2009). An MUAC measurement of between 11.5 and 12.5 cm classifies a child between the ages of six and 60 months as moderately acutely malnourished (WHO 2013; WHO and UNICEF 2009).

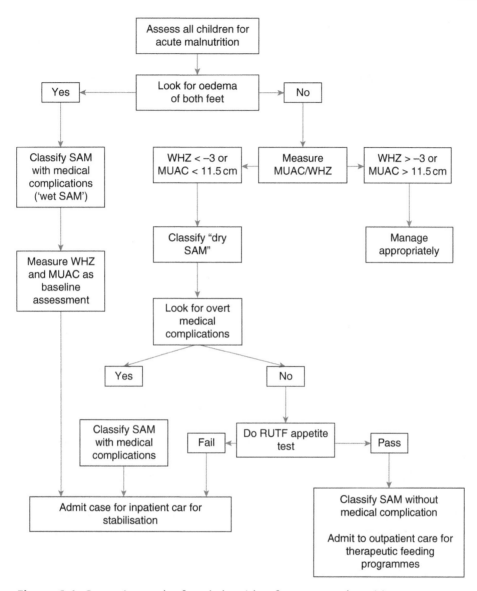

Figure 6.4: Screening and referral algorithm for acute malnutrition.

WFH and WFL Z-scores are used to identify SAM (WHO 2013). A WFH < −3 is associated with a greatly increased risk of death (WHO 2006), which is why the cut-off is set at −3 SD (WHO and UNICEF 2009). MUAC can be used interchangeably to identify children with SAM (WHO 2013). An MUAC measurement of 11.5 cm is used to identify SAM, and MUAC < 11.5 cm and WHZ < −3 identify a similar prevalence of SAM in the field (WHO and UNICEF 2009)

Children are identified in the community by trained community health workers by assessing mid-upper arm circumference and the presence of bilateral pitting oedema. Children 6–59 months old with

MUAC < 12.5 cm and any degree of oedema are referred immediately to a treatment centre for a full assessment for SAM. The full assessment includes plotting and interpreting weight for height, an examination of oedema, a clinical examination for IMCI danger signs and an appetite test. Children with an MUAC < 11.5 cm or WFH < –3 or severe bilateral pitting oedema presenting with medical complications or poor appetite are treated as inpatients. Children without medical complications, pass an appetite test and are alert can be treated as outpatients (WHO 2013).

6.4 Clinical Signs of Malnutrition

Anthropometry (measuring the human body) is the 'gold standard' for determining nutritional status, but it is still important to be able to recognise the signs and symptoms of malnutrition in the field, in order to make the best decisions for intervention quickly.

Emaciation/Wasting is the name given to the condition when people are so thin that they look skeletal. The cheek bones and temples become very pronounced, and the fontanel on the top of the head is often indented in infants (also commonly caused by dehydration that is associated with malnutrition). The arms and legs may appear very thin, and ribs may easily be visible through the skin.

Oedema is fluid retention and occurs frequently in severely malnourished children. Children with oedema will have puffy, swollen feet, hands or face. Test for oedema by pressing gently into the skin. If your finger leaves an imprint or pit, the child has oedema. Children with bilateral (on both sides) pitting oedema must be referred to the hospital immediately.

Hair becomes very brittle and weak. It is pulled out easily and often looks patchy. It may also lose some of its colour and appear orange.

Skin is marked by dry patches that might be red and bleeding in very bad cases. This is known as dermatitis.

The mouth might present with painful sores at the corners of the lips, known as angular stomatosis, which is caused by a weakened immune system and vitamin B deficiency. The tongue might be pale or covered in a white or red 'fur', which is a sign of oral infection caused by a weakened immune system. Mouth problems can cause appetite problems, which worsen malnutrition.

Loss of appetite is a common complication of starvation. Ask the mother or caregiver how the child is eating to evaluate appetite or perform an appetite test using a ready-to-use therapeutic food (RUTF). Malnourished children with a WFH Z-score below the –3 line, or an MUAC of less than 11.5 cm, as well as loss of appetite, must be referred to the hospital immediately.

6.5 Pathophysiology of Acute Malnutrition

This section compares metabolism in healthy, well-nourished people with metabolism in malnourished ones. It details how glycogen stores, then adipose tissue, and finally protein stores are catabolised to provide fuel for the body during starvation. It also describes changes in fluid and electrolyte status.

Marasmic infants have a greater gut permeability than well-nourished infants (Behrens et al. 1987). Villous atrophy is present and therefore lactase enzymes usually present in the villi are absent. This results in the absorption of lactose that is only partially hydrolysed and therefore excreted in the urine at higher rates than in well-nourished children (Behrens et al. 1987). This malabsorption may help to explain the link between malnutrition and diarrhoeal disease.

The term 'protein energy malnutrition' referring to kwashiorkor and marasmus places emphasis on protein and energy deficits in the development of these conditions; however, the pathophysiology of acute malnutrition is not limited to protein or caloric deficiency. Acute malnutrition is a complex condition and involves a range of macro- and micronutrients and multiple organ systems.

6.5.1 Metabolism in Healthy People

Human fuel reserves are composed of glycogen, one-third of which is located in the liver and the remainder in the muscles; protein stores in the muscles and vital organs and triglycerides in the adipose tissue.

Approximately two hours after a meal, blood glucose begins to reduce, and blood glucose is supplemented by the glycogen stores (Figure 6.5). At this stage, there is little synthesis of triglycerides. Four hours after a meal, blood glucose drops further, and triglycerides are mobilised as the primary fuel source for the muscles and liver. Proteins are degraded to glucose to supply energy to the brain.

6.5.2 Metabolism in Acute Malnutrition

In states of acute malnutrition, there are low serum concentrations of albumin, free amino acids, propionyl (C3) carnitine, and other by-products of branched chain amino acid metabolism (Freemark 2015). This suggests that muscle stores are initially protected.

In the early stages of starvation (Figures 6.6 and 6.7), blood glucose concentrations drop, resulting in a reduction of serum insulin concentrations and increased concentrations of glucagon. Raised growth

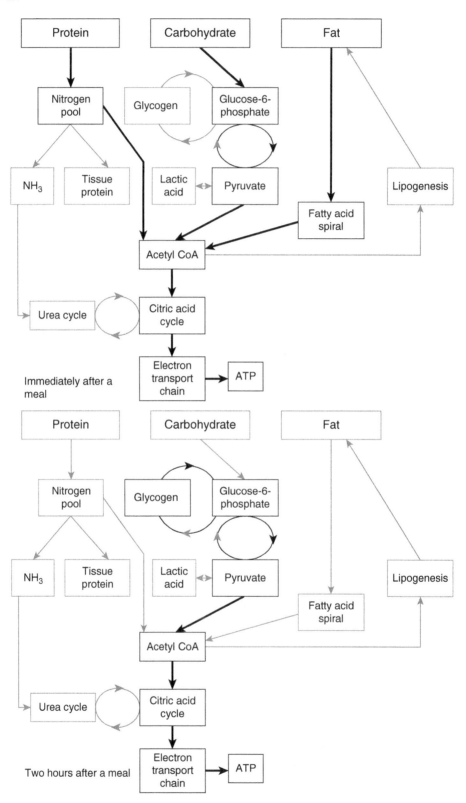

Figure 6.5: Metabolism of substrates following a meal in well-nourished individuals.

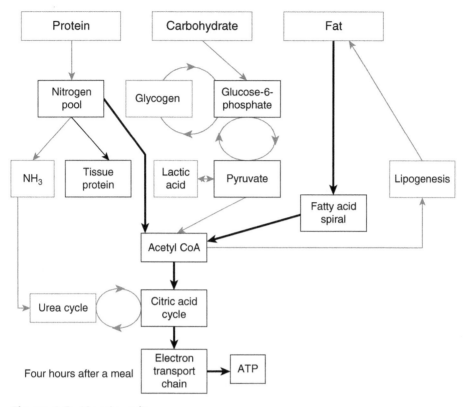

Figure 6.5: (Continued)

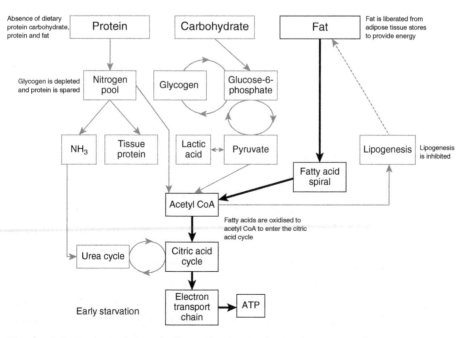

Figure 6.6: Favoured metabolic pathways in the early stages of starvation.

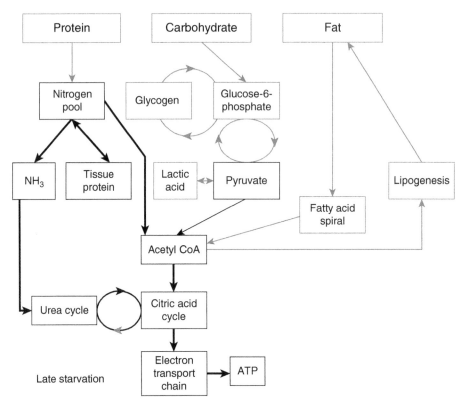

Figure 6.7: Preferred metabolic pathways in late starvation.

hormone concentrations and lower rates of insulin secretion result in hepatic glucose production and gluconeogenesis, with a simultaneous increased rate of lipolysis and reduced rate of proteolysis. Triglycerides in adipose tissue are catabolised to free fatty acids and glycerol, which are converted to ketone bodies (McCray et al. 2009). Adipose reserves are depleted quickly in favour of lean muscle tissue and vital organ tissue as an adaptation to starvation (Briend et al. 2015).

The stress hormone cortisol is stimulated by anxiety, infection, low blood glucose and states of starvation. Cortisol acts on the liver, muscle and adipose tissues. It stimulates increased release of triglycerides from adipose tissue. The fatty acids from the triglycerides are used as a fuel source for the tissues, and glycerol is used for gluconeogenesis in the liver (Nelson and Cox 2015). An increased turnover of cell membranes and fatty acids is observed in acute malnutrition (Fondu et al. 1980).

There are raised serum levels of non-esterified fatty acids, ketones and even-chained acylglycerides, indicating accelerated fat metabolism or lipolysis (Bartz et al. 2014; Freemark 2015). Once the fat reserves have been depleted, the degradation of essential protein stores begins, including organs such as the heart and liver (Nelson and Cox 2015).

Adipose tissue plays an important role in thermoregulation. Depleted fat stores in acutely malnourished children alongside reduced brown fat levels result in poor insulation and heat generation (Brooke 1972). Observations of acutely malnourished children show that their body temperature follows changes in ambient temperature, suggesting a diminished ability to generate body heat (Brooke 1972). It is thought that basal metabolism is reduced as an adaptation to prevent excess caloric expenditure, resulting in lower heat generation (Brooke 1972).

6.5.3 Micronutrient Deficiency

Micronutrient deficiencies of selenium, vitamin A, zinc, iron and copper are common in acutely malnourished children (Weisstaub et al. 2008). Zinc and vitamin A deficiencies affect immune system function and the structure and function of mucosal membranes (Bhan et al. 2003). Zinc supplementation reduces the incidence of diarrhoea and pneumonia, and promotes growth (Zinc Investigators Collaborative Group 1999). Hospitalised children with acute malnutrition respond well to copper, iron and zinc supplementation according to WHO protocols (Weisstaub et al. 2008)

Essential fatty acid (EFA) deficiency may be related to some of the symptoms observed in acute malnutrition (Smit et al. 2004). EFAs are involved in maintaining healthy skin, immune response, growth and brain development. Acute malnutrition often presents with scaly dermatitis, disruption to linear growth and cognitive developmental delay. A reduced intake of EFAs amongst sufferers of acute malnutrition may result in EFA deficiency, which negatively affects fatty acid absorption and transport (Smit et al. 2004). EFA deficiency may also result in reduced nutrient absorption and poorer calorie utilisation via structural changes to mitochondrial membranes, in turn worsening malnutrition (Smit et al. 2004).

6.5.4 Fluid and Hydration

Acute malnutrition is associated with some changes in fluid and electrolyte balance that can have fatal consequences if not managed correctly. Children who are acutely malnourished have excess body sodium, although plasma sodium concentrations are low (Ashworth et al. 2003). Potassium and magnesium deficiencies are usually present and in combination with excess sodium are partly responsible for oedema. Dehydration is common in acute malnutrition and is related to shock and lethargy seen as clinical signs of malnutrition. It is difficult to assess hydration status in severely malnourished children. Low blood volume can coexist with oedema. Oedema seen in severely malnourished children is a result of low serum albumin, increased cortisol and inability to activate antidiuretic hormone (Dipasquale et al. 2020).

6.5.5 Understanding Refeeding Syndrome as Part of Acute Malnutrition

Starvation results in higher rates of gluconeogenesis from amino acids. Members of the B vitamin group are depleted as they act as co-enzymes in these reactions. Eventually, there is a depletion of substrates.

When refeeding begins, gluconeogenesis stops, and instead of catabolic reactions, metabolism shifts to anabolism. Carbohydrates ingested during refeeding stimulate insulin secretion. A major role of (Figure 6.8) insulin is to allow glucose to enter the cells.

Fluid shifts in the human body rely on the polarity of water molecules. The oxygen atom of a water molecule is larger and heavier than the two hydrogen atoms, resulting in more electronegativity around the oxygen atom – the electrons spend more time around this atom, creating a slightly negative charge. Simultaneously, a slightly positive charge is found around the hydrogen atoms (Figure 6.9).

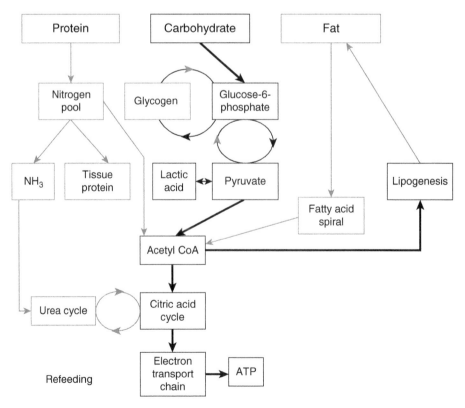

Figure 6.8: Metabolic changes as a result of refeeding.

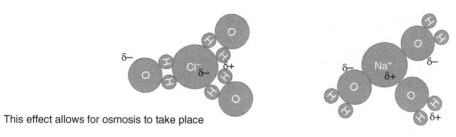

This effect allows for osmosis to take place

Figure 6.9: Polarity of water molecules and interactions with the electrolytes.

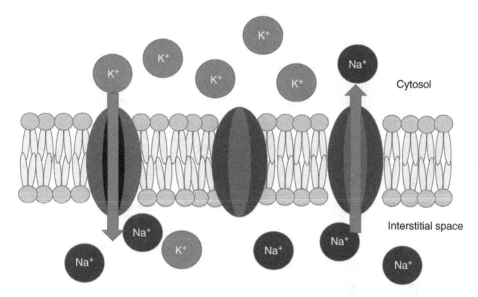

Figure 6.10: The cell's neutral charge is maintained by electrolytes leaving and entering the cytosol for the interstitial space.

The electrolytes are positive cations and negative anions, and the main electrolytes involved in human physiology are sodium and potassium (cations) and chloride (anion). The cations and anions balance the neutral charge of cells; if sodium (Na+) leaves the cell for the interstitial space, K+ enters the cell to maintain the neutral charge (Figure 6.10).

As water molecules are polar, the electrolytes attract water to themselves, and as they pass in and out of cells, pulling water along with them. This allows osmosis to take place, maintaining cell turgor.

During refeeding, metabolism switches from catabolism to anabolism (Figure 6.11). Insulin is the major anabolic hormone and is secreted in response to rising glucose levels from digestion.

The electrolytes are not the only molecules with this capacity – water will also follow glucose in and out of cells. When refeeding starts and glucose enters cells, water follows. Glucose enters cells via active transport through membrane proteins that rely on a change in electrochemical

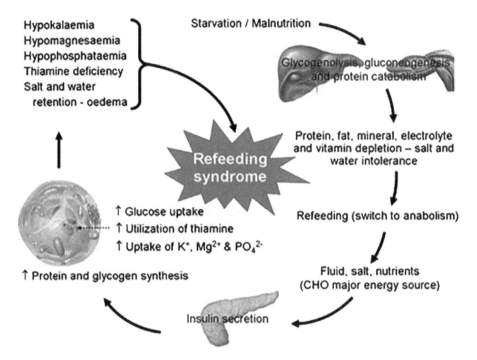

Figure 6.11: The refeeding syndrome.

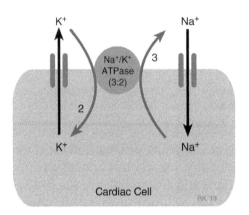

Figure 6.12: Electrolyte activity in cardiac cells.

potential difference to move glucose against the concentration gradient. This is achieved by moving sodium from a high concentration to a low concentration – glucose and sodium enter the cell together along with water. The new high concentration of sodium in the cell activates the Na K ATPase pump, and sodium is pumped out of the cell and replaced with potassium to maintain the charge (Figure 6.12). In severe malnutrition, this can rapidly result in hypokalaemia.

Thiamine is a B vitamin and co-enzyme involved in glycolysis (Figure 6.13). Glucose is converted to pyruvate in the first stage of glycolysis. The conversion of pyruvate to acetyl co-A requires the

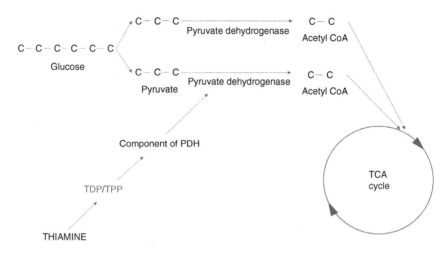

Figure 6.13: Role of thiamine in the conversion of pyruvate to acetyl coA.

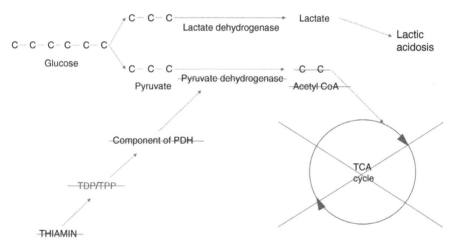

Figure 6.14: The fate of pyruvate is lactate when thiamine is depleted.

co-enzyme pyruvate dehydrogenase, which is derived from thiamine. When there is enough thiamine available, pyruvate is converted to acetyl co-A and enters the TCA cycle to generate ATP.

However, when the body is depleted of thiamine, pyruvate dehydrogenase cannot be produced, and instead of conversion of pyruvate to acetyl Co-A, pyruvate is converted into lactate, which results in lactic acidosis (Figure 6.14).

The combination of hypokalaemia and lactic acidosis is responsible for the features of the refeeding syndrome, including heart failure and oedema. Therefore, careful introduction of foods, fluids and electrolytes and replenishment of B vitamins are required to prevent mortality in starving patients.

6.5.5.1 Clinical Management of Severe Acute Malnutrition

Children with an MUAC < 11.5 cm or WFH < −3 or severe bilateral pitting oedema presenting with medical complications or poor appetite are treated as inpatients using the WHO 10 Steps to Treating Severe Acute Malnutrition protocol. Children without medical complications, pass an appetite test and are alert can be treated as outpatients.

WHO guidelines on the management of SAM are largely based on expert opinion (Tickell and Denno 2016). The WHO recognises that the evidence base for current recommendations is poor due to a lack of recent randomised controlled trials and observational studies (WHO 2013). Indirect evidence from other populations or treatment methods informs guidelines where direct evidence is not available (WHO 2013).

Children identified with SAM should have a full medical examination screen for clinical complications and appetite (WHO 2013). An appetite test takes place, and children are assessed for severe oedema, medical complications and the presence of Integrated Management of Childhood Illness danger signs (WHO 2013). Failing the appetite test and presenting with complications or danger signs mean that the child should be treated as an inpatient. Uncomplicated cases with a good appetite can be treated in the community (WHO 2013).

As malnutrition is a risk factor for infection, children with SAM often present with infection. However, symptoms of infection such as fever are often absent. Hypoglycaemia and hypothermia occurring together are signs of infection in acutely malnourished children (Ashworth et al. 2003).

Common biochemical abnormalities in severely malnourished children include low urea, hypoprotienaemia, hypokalaemia, hypophosphataemia, hypomagnesaemia, hypoglycaemia and anaemia (Golden 2002).

The guidelines for treating inpatient malnutrition include 10 steps as general principles for routine care (Ashworth et al. 2003). These steps are divided into an initial stabilisation phase and a longer rehabilitation phase. The 10 steps are to treat or prevent hypoglycaemia, treat or prevent hypothermia, treat or prevent dehydration, correct electrolyte imbalance, treat or prevent infection, correct micronutrient deficiencies, start cautious feeding, achieve catch-up growth, provide sensory stimulation and emotional support and finally to prepare for follow-up after recovery (Ashworth et al. 2003).

Micronutrient deficiency is corrected with vitamin A, folic acid, zinc and copper supplements. Iron supplements are withheld until the child has begun gaining weight as they increase the risk of infection in the initial phase (Ashworth et al. 2003).

Cautious feeding is required in the stabilisation phase due to reduced homeostatic capacity and poor physiological state (Ashworth et al. 2003).

Caloric and protein targets are met using the milk-based starter formula F-75, which contains 75 kcal and 0.9 g protein per 100 ml.

The return of the child's appetite approximately a week into the stabilisation phase is the signal to change to the rehabilitation phase (Ashworth et al. 2003). The F-75 formula is replaced with F-100 (100 kcal, 2.9 g protein per 100 ml) to provide more energy and protein for rebuilding tissues. Volumes of F-100 are gradually increased per feed and are often used in combination with modified porridges and family foods (Ashworth et al. 2003).

SAM patients are considered recovered when they have achieved a -1 SD weight for length score (Ashworth et al. 2003). It is likely they will have a low weight for age Z-score due to stunting (Ashworth et al. 2003). Discharge from hospital should include training the child's carer to continue giving frequent nutrient and energy dense foods as well as structured play therapy, arrangements should be made for follow-up, booster immunizations given and vitamin A supplements must be given every six months (Ashworth et al. 2003).

Children with SAM should have a full medical examination screen for clinical complications such as severe oedema, medical complications and the presence of Integrated Management of Childhood Illness danger signs (WHO 2013). This assessment should include an assessment of whether the child is breastfeeding and taking the usual diet, the current oral intake of the child. History of diarrhoea and vomiting should be assessed, identifying whether diarrhoea is watery or bloody. History of TB or TB contact, HIV infection or suspected HIV infection should be assessed. The child should be assessed for oedema, shock and lethargy and hypothermia. These children may also present with signs of vitamin A deficiency, mouth ulcers and pallor (Golden 2002).

An appetite test should be performed according to WHO protocols (WHO 2013). Failing an appetite test or presenting with complications or danger signs, the child should be treated as an inpatient. Uncomplicated cases with a good appetite can be treated in the community (WHO 2013).

6.5.6 The WHO 10 Steps

The guidelines for treating inpatient malnutrition are presented as 10 steps as general principles for routine care (Ashworth et al. 2003). Steps are divided into an initial stabilisation phase and a longer rehabilitation phase (Figure 6.15).

The 10 steps are to:

1. Treat or prevent hypoglycaemia
2. Treat or prevent hypothermia
3. Treat or prevent dehydration

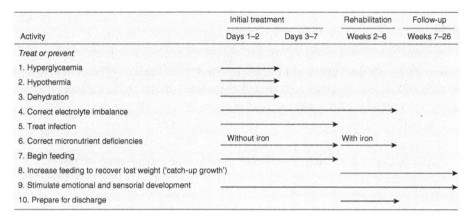

	Initial treatment		Rehabilitation	Follow-up
Activity	Days 1–2	Days 3–7	Weeks 2–6	Weeks 7–26
Treat or prevent				
1. Hyperglycaemia	⟶			
2. Hypothermia	⟶			
3. Dehydration	⟶			
4. Correct electrolyte imbalance	⟶			
5. Treat infection	⟶			
6. Correct micronutrient deficiencies	Without iron ⟶		With iron ⟶	
7. Begin feeding	⟶			
8. Increase feeding to recover lost weight ('catch-up growth')			⟶	
9. Stimulate emotional and sensorial development	⟶			
10. Prepare for discharge			⟶	

Figure 6.15: Timing of the WHO 10 Steps for treating severe acute malnutrition.

4. Correct electrolyte imbalance
5. Treat or prevent infection
6. Correct micronutrient deficiencies
7. Start cautious feeding
8. Achieve catch-up growth
9. Provide sensory stimulation and emotional support
10. Prepare for follow-up after recovery (Ashworth et al. 2003)

Step 1: Treat or prevent hypoglycaemia. Hypoglycaemia was associated with a 2.74-fold increase in the risk of mortality amongst children with SAM in a stabilisation centre in the Gedeo Zone (Girum et al. 2017). The IMCI danger signs include loss of consciousness and convulsions, which along with lethargy, limpness and low body temperature may be signs of hypoglycaemia. Sweating may be absent due to dehydration. Treatment should begin while the child is being admitted for care (does not need to wait for admission) and should include small frequent feeds and treatment of infections (Golden 2002).

Step 2: Treat or prevent hypothermia. Studies usually use a body temperature of 35 °C as the cut-off value for hypothermia (Brooke 1972; Talbert et al. 2009). In response to reduced caloric intake, metabolism is reduced in acutely malnourished children, resulting in lower heat production. Hypothermia is a serious complication of SAM (Brooke 1972). Altered temperature amongst SAM patients younger than five years was associated with an increased mortality risk seven times higher than those without changes to their temperature (Girum et al. 2017). The WHO recommends regular 2–4 hourly temperature measurements of children being treated for SAM, while they are in the 'stabilisation phase' of treatment (World Health Organisation 2011). However, this number of body temperature measurements may not be feasible in resource-poor settings where clinical staff and equipment are limited (Mole et al. 2012). Furthermore, it has been suggested that hypothermia is not a common occurrence (Mole et al. 2012; Talbert et al. 2009) amongst children admitted to the hospital with SAM and that the timing of hypothermia does not coincide with clinical deterioration, even though the mortality rate amongst children with a temperature below 35 °C is higher (Talbert et al. 2009). Talbert et al. (2009) have suggested that other mortality risk factors should be prioritised over monitoring body temperature where few staff are available. Body temperature appears to respond rapidly to refeeding (within two hours); therefore, frequent feeding is recommended to maintain body temperature (Brooke 1972). Alternative temperature monitoring methods may also potentially assist where there is insufficient staff to carry out measurements with a thermometer, such as ThermoSpots, which are stickers that change colour to indicate drops in temperature and show a good sensitivity and specificity compared with the gold standard rectal temperature (Mole et al. 2012). Practical guidance for treating and preventing hypothermia amongst these children is to keep them in a warm room (25–30 °C) without draughts. Washing should be kept to the minimum necessary, and children should be washed with warm water wherever possible. The child should be dried immediately (Golden 2002). Feeding frequently can assist with maintaining heat generation through thermogenesis and should take place at daytime and night-time. Clinicians should avoid medical examinations that leave the child cold (Golden 2002).

Step 3: Treat or prevent dehydration. Dehydration in severe malnutrition does not present as in other children, so normal signs may be absent. It should be assumed that any severely malnourished child with watery diarrhoea is dehydrated. Clinicians should check the history of the child to determine whether there has been frequent, watery diarrhoea or a history of not passing urine (Golden 2002).

Dehydration in acutely malnourished children with complications must be corrected with ReSoMal. This is because standard rehydration solutions and IV lines increase the risk of cardiac fluid overload due to their high sodium content. The recommended rate and volume of ReSoMal for rehydrating acutely malnourished children is 5 ml/kg/h for four hours, gradually increasing to 5–10 ml/kg/h for the next four hours, and finally replacing ReSoMal with the F-75 formula. During rehydration, clinicians should monitor the child's pulse, respiratory rate, urine frequency, stool and vomit frequency. Clinicians may see return of tears, moist mouth, sunken fontanelle and return of skin turgor; however, many malnourished children will not exhibit these changes.

6.5.7 ReSoMal Recipe

2 l cooled boiled water
1 l packet WHO ORS (3.5 g NaCl, 2.9 g trisodium citrate dehydrate, 1.5 g KCl and 20 g glucose)
50 g sugar
40 ml electrolyte/mineral solution

Frequent assessments should take place during rehydration – initially every 30 minutes and then hourly after the first two hours.

Step 4: Correct electrolyte imbalance. Potassium and magnesium deficiencies are present amongst children with SAM. Low plasma sodium may mask high body sodium levels. Electrolyte imbalances along with bradycardia in acutely malnourished children predispose them to arrhythmias (Dipasquale et al. 2020). Electrolyte imbalances are also a contributing factor to impaired ventilatory responses to hypoxia (Dipasquale et al. 2020).

Step 5: Treat or prevent infection. Inflammatory responses are diminished in SAM; therefore, acutely malnourished children may not present with signs of infection and may be assumed to have infections (Golden 2002).

The immune system is impaired by acute malnutrition. The thymus, lymph nodes and tonsils are atrophied in SAM, and CD4 and CD8 T-cells are reduced in number and function (Dipasquale et al. 2020). Therefore, the risk of infection is higher amongst these children.

Step 6: Correct micronutrient deficiency

Anaemia doubles the risk of mortality amongst children with SAM (Girum et al. 2017). Micronutrient deficiency is corrected with vitamin A, folic acid zinc and copper supplements. Iron supplements are withheld until the child has begun gaining weight. This is because iron supplementation increases the risk of infection in the initial phase (Ashworth et al. 2003). Haemoglobin should only be measured at admission, and anaemia should be corrected with transfusion at this point only. Transfusions should not be given after haemodilution takes place when rehydration and correction of electrolyte imbalance begin, putting the child at high risk of heart failure (Golden 2002).

Step 7: Start cautious feeding. Malnourished children present with villous atrophy and pancreatic atrophy which cause malabsorption (Dipasquale et al. 2020).

Cautious feeding should start on admission. The aim of this stage is to meet requirements for maintaining physiological processes, but no more as the child will be in a poor physiological state. The child should be provided small, frequent meals. Feed should have the low-lactose milk-based starter formula F-75 (Ashworth et al. 2003) that provides 75 kcal, 0.9 g protein per 100 ml. Children should not gain weight during this phase, and children with oedema are likely to lose weight as the oedema subsides.

Step 8: Achieve catch-up growth. Once the child's appetite has returned, treatment can change from stabilisation to achieving catch-up growth (Ashworth et al. 2003). This may occur after a few days amongst children without oedema and approximately a week into treatment in complicated cases. The F-75 formula is changed to F-100, which provides 100 kcal and 2.9 g protein per 100 ml. This higher energy and protein formula and gradually increased volume of feeds in combination with reintroduction of modified porridges and other foods provides the nutrients required for growth and rehabilitating tissues (Ashworth et al. 2003).

Step 9: Provide sensory stimulation and emotional support. Brain development is negatively impacted by SAM (Prado and Dewey 2014). Structural changes occur in the brain as a result of acute malnutrition, including reduced numbers of neurons and synapses (Dipasquale et al. 2020). Stimulation should focus on activities that stimulate a child's mental development, and the mother should be involved in activities and encouraged to talk to and play with her child. Providing treatment increases scores in academic and language tests in the months and years following recovery; however, recovered children with SAM do not perform as well as well-nourished controls, suggesting that some long-term damage to cognitive skills is inevitable (Grantham-McGregor et al. 1980). Similar results were seen for fine motor skills (Grantham-McGregor et al. 1980). Results from intervention studies show that there is no difference in emotional outcomes amongst recovered SAM children and non-malnourished controls, suggesting that intervention can be effective (Grantham-McGregor et al. 1980). However, more research is needed on psychomotor and sensory stimulation amongst children with SAM as very few high-quality studies are available (Daniel et al. 2017).

Step 10: Prepare for follow-up after recovery. The final step is to prepare discharge plans for the child. Children are considered recovered from SAM when they have achieved WFH < –1 (Ashworth et al. 2003). It should be noted that weight for age is likely to be low due to stunting (Ashworth et al. 2003). Discharge plans from the hospital should include arrangements for follow-up, booster immunisations and plans for vitamin A supplementation every six months. Carers of the child should be trained on giving frequent nutrient and energy dense foods and structured play (Ashworth et al. 2003).

6.5.7.1 Community-Based Management of Acute Malnutrition (CMAM)

The community-based management of acute malnutrition (CMAM) model was first developed by Valid International and the FANTA project. It has been widely adopted in low- and middle-income regions to treat uncomplicated SAM.

The WHO inpatient model for treating SAM is effective in reducing case mortalities. However, resource-poor environments are unable to meet demands for skilled staff (Collins et al. 2006). Barriers to successful treatment in resource-poor areas include inadequate feeding, poor management of rehydration and infection, lack of resources and the lack of knowledge and motivated staff (Puoane et al. 2001).

The Tamil Nadu Integrated Nutrition Project was a prototype of community-based management of acute malnutrition which started in 1980. This intervention made use of growth monitoring and short-term supplementary feeding to improve the nutritional status of children. Local women were recruited to assist with growth monitoring. This programme proved to be cost-effective and demonstrated that longer-term feeding was not required to improve the nutritional status. Improved child feeding practices can be sustained through nutrition education (Skolnik 2012).

Triaging SAM cases with complications for hospital care while treating uncomplicated acute malnutrition in the community reduces inpatient caseloads while increasing coverage rates (Collins et al. 2006). Children with SAM and good appetite can be managed as ambulatory patients by infection treatment and the use of RUTF or appropriately formulated home diets. Optimal management of children with moderate acute malnutrition (namely use of RUTF versus specialised home-prepared diets) is being investigated to develop simple, effective and affordable dietary regimens (Brown et al. 2009).

6.5.8 The CMAM Model

The CMAM model was developed by Valid International and Concern Worldwide. The decentralised nature of CMAM allows programmes to reach even highly dispersed rural populations in harsh environments. The advantages of the CMAM model are that it maximises coverage and access to services, allows for the early detection of malnutrition, provides care that is appropriate for patients and provides prolonged care and integration into child health and social services.

Outpatient therapeutic programmes bring the service of management of SAM closer to the community (Yebyo et al. 2013). Decentralised health facilities mean that children with acute malnutrition can be managed at home in the catchment area of a health centre or health post. Services rendered at the decentralised sites include screening and growth monitoring, provision of RUTF and vitamin A and deworming treatment (Yebyo et al. 2013). Anthropometry is often monitored monthly while RUTF is given in weekly rations (Collins et al. 2006).

6.5.9 Ready-to-Use Therapeutic Foods (RUTF) and Ready-to-Use Supplementary Foods (RUSF)

Ready-to-use supplementary foods and RUTFs are used in the treatment of acute malnutrition in hospitals and the community. These foods are found in the form of milk formulas, porridges and pastes. Ideally, they need to meet the energy and protein specifications of F75 or F100 formulas and should be shelf stable for long periods of time, acceptable to the consumer and safe.

Variations of supplementary foods for treating moderate acute malnutrition are an area of active research. Variations need to meet international energy and protein specifications for the management of infants and young children with moderate acute malnutrition and are often developed with locally sourced or functional ingredients. Veldman et al. (2020) substituted the corn in a fortified corn–soya blend porridge with enzyme-active sorghum malt. Walsh et al. (2018) investigated a legume-based, lactose-free RUSF. As SAM is associated with changes in intestinal mucosa integrity and diarrhoea, as well as transient lactose intolerance, the researchers hypothesised that lactose-free, fermentable carbohydrate-based feeds may help to reduce the incidence of lactose intolerance-related diarrhoea and improve mucosal integrity (Walsh et al. 2018).

Isanaka et al. (2019) compared the cost-effectiveness of four RUSF products in treating moderate acute malnutrition. They compared a commercial RUSF product, fortified local legume and cereal blend, a corn–soya blend, and locally milled flour made up of millet, beans, oil, sugar and micronutrient powder to no treatment for MAM. It was found that the commercial RUSF reduces the risk of death by 15.5% compared with no treatment. There was a 12.7% reduction in the risk of death for the corn–soya blend, a reduced risk of 11.9% for the fortified legume and cereal blend and a 10.3% reduction in mortality risk for the locally milled flour (Isanaka et al. 2019). Treating MAM with RUSF is a cost-effective method. The incremented cost-effectiveness ratio was US$9821 per death averted or US$347 per disability-adjusted life year (DALY) for treatment with RUSF compared with no treatment (Isanaka et al. 2019).

Shen et al. (2019) compared four isocaloric rations of ready-to-use supplementary food for cost-effectiveness – corn–soya blend plus with oil; corn–soya whey blend with oil; and super cereal plus; and RUSF. The prices of the treatments ranged from US$86 for RUSF to US$94 for super cereal. The cost per recovered child was US$137 to US$149. It was found that crude cost-effectiveness to treat MAM considering only implementer costs was similar across the four supplementary foods. The product and international freight costs were the biggest drivers for cost-effectiveness (Shen et al. 2019). Cost-effectiveness may be useful for decision makers when deciding on treatment for acute malnutrition (Langlois et al. 2019).

There has been a high rate of relapse into malnutrition observed amongst children successfully treated for SAM within one year (Chang et al. 2013). Seasonal patterns of food security and adverse clinical outcomes may be factors related to relapse (Chang et al. 2013). It was found that treatment with soya- or whey-based RUSF was more effective than corn blend or milk and oil (Chang et al. 2013). Importantly, children treated for MAM in the community remain vulnerable to relapse after treatment.

References

Ali, W.A., Ayub, A., and Hussain, H. (2015). Prevalence and associated risk factors of under nutrition among children aged 6–59 months in internally displaced persons of Jalozai camp, district Nowshera, Khybes Pakhtunkhwa. *J. Ayub Med. Coll. Abbottabad* 23 (7): 556–559.

Ashworth, A., Khanum, S., Jackson, A., and Schofield, C. (2003). *Guidelines for the Inpatient Treatment of Severely Malnourished Children*. Geneva: World Health Organisation.

Bartz, S., Mody, A., Hornik, C. et al. (2014). Severe acute malnutrition in childhood: hormonal and metabolic status at presentation, response to treatment, and predictors of mortality. *J. Endocrinol. Metab.* 99 (6): 2128–2137.

Behrens, R.H., Lunn, P.G., Northropp, C.A. et al. (1987). Factors affecting the integrity of the intestinal mucosa of Gambian children. *Am. J. Clin. Nutr.* 45: 1433–1431.

Bhan, M.K., Bhandari, N., and Bahl, R. (2003). Management of the severely malnourished child: perspective from developing countries. *Br. Med. J.* 326: 146.

Bhutta, Z.A., Akseer, N., Kets, E.C. et al. (2020). How countries can reduce child stunting at scale: lessons from exemplar countries. *Am. J. Clin. Nutr.* 112 (S2): 894S–904S.

Black, R.E., Victoria, C.G., Walker, S.P. et al. (2013). Maternal and child nutrition and overweight in low-income and middle-income countries. *Lancet Series Maternal Child Nutr.* 1: 1–25.

Briend, A., Khara, T., and Dolan, C. (2015). Wasting and stunting- similarities and differences. Policy and programmatic implications. *Food and Nutrit. Bullet.* 36 (S1): https://doi.org/10.1177%2F15648265150361S103.

Brooke, O. (1972). Influence of malnutrition on the body temperature of children. *Br. Med. J.* 1: 331–332.

Brown, K.H., Nyirandutiye, D.H., and Jungjohan, S. (2009). Management of children with acute malnutrition in resource-poor settings. *Nat. Rev. Endocrinol.* 5: 597–603.

Chang, C.Y., Trehan, I., Wang, R.J. et al. (2013). Children successfully treated for moderate acute malnutrition remain at high risk for malnutrition and death in subsequent year after recovery. *J. Nutr.* 143 (2): 215–220.

Chowdhury, R., Sinha, B., Adhikary, M. et al. (2013). Developing models to predict stunting among 6-59 months children in a slum in Kolkata. *Indian J. Community Health* 25 (3): 251–256.

Collins, S., Dent, N., Binns, P. et al. (2006). Management of severe acute malnutrition in children. *Lancet* 368: 1992–2000.

Daniel, A.I., Bandsma, R.H., Lytvyn, L. et al. (2017). Psychological stimulation interventions for children with severe acute malnutrition: a systematic review. *J. Glob. Health* 7 (1): 010405.

Dipasquale, V., Cucinotta, U., and Romano, C. (2020). Acute malnutrition in children: pathophysiology, clinical effects and treatment. *Nutrients* 12 (2413): https://doi.org/10.3390/nu12082413.

Fink, G. and Rockers, P.C. (2014). Childhood growth, schooling and cognitive development: further evidence from the Young Lives study. *Am. J. Clin. Nutr.* 100 (1): 182–188.

Fondu, P., Mozez, N., Neve, P. et al. (1980). The erythrocyte membrane disturbances in protein-energy malnutrition: nature and mechanisms. *Br. J. Haematol.* 44 (4): 605–618.

Freemark, M. (2015). Metabolomics in nutrition research: biomarkers predicting mortality in children with severe acute malnutrition. *Food Nutr. Bull.* 36 (1): S88–S92.

Gachau, S., Irimu, G., Ayieko, P. et al. (2018). Prevalence, outcome and quality of care among children hospitalised with severe acute malnutrition in Kenyan hospitals: a multi-site observational study. *PLoS One* 13 (5): e0197607.

Girum, T., Kote, M., Tariku, B., and Bekele, H. (2017). Survival status and predictors of mortality among severely malnourished children <5 years of age admitted to stabilisation centres in Gedeo zone: a retrospective cohort study. *Ther. Clin. Risk Manag.* 13: 101–110.

Golden, M.H.N. (2002). Severe malnutrition: appearing. In: *International Child Health Care: A Practical Manual for Hospitals Worldwide* (ed. D. Southall, B. Coulter, C. Ronald, et al.). London: BMJ Books.

Grantham-McGregor, S., Stewart, M., Powell, C., and Schofield, W.N. (1980). Stimulation and mental development of malnourished infants. *Lancet* 1 (89): https://doi.org/10.1016/S0140-6736(80)90509-7.

Haddinott, J., Alderman, H., Behrman, J.R. et al. (2013). The economic rationale for investing in stunting reduction. *Matern. Child Nutr.* 9 (S2): 69–82.

Isanaka, S., Barnhart, D.A., McDonald, C.M. et al. (2019). Cost-effectiveness of community-based screening and treatment of moderate acute malnutrition in Mali. *BMJ Glob. Health* 4: e001227.

Keino, S., Plasqui, G., Ettyang, G., and den Borne, V. (2014). Determinants of stunting and overweight among young children and adolescents in sub-Saharan Africa. Determinants of stunting and overweight among young children and adolescents in sub-Saharan Africa. *Food and Nutrit. Bullet.* 35 (2): https://doi.org/10.1177%2F156482651403500203.

Kimani-Murage, E.W. (2013). Exploring the paradox: double burden of malnutrition in rural South Africa. *Glob. Health Action* 6: 193–205.

Langlois, B., Griswold, S., Suri, D. et al. (2019). Comparative effectiveness of four specialised nutritious food products for treatment of moderate acute malnutrition in Sierra Leone. *Curr. Dev. Nutr.* 3 (S1): 918.

Makiwane, M. (2010). The child support grant and teenage childbearing in South Africa. *Develop. South Africa* 27 (2): 193–204.

Maluccio, J.A., Hoddinott, J., Behrman, J.R. et al. (2009). The impact of improving nutrition during early childhood on education among Guatemalan adults. *Econ. J.* 119 (537): 734–763.

Mamabolo, R.L., Alberts, M., Steyn, N.P. et al. (2005). Prevalence and determinants of stunting and overweight in 3-year old black South African children residing in the Central Region of Limpopo Province, South Africa. *Public Health Nutr.* 8 (5): 501–508.

Mata, L. (1992). Diarrhoeal disease as a cause of malnutrition. *Am. J. Trop. Med. Hyg.* 47 (S1): 16–27.

McCray, S., Walker, S., and Parish, C.R. (2009). Much ado about refeeding. *Pract. Gastroenterol.* 26–44.

Mole, T.B., Kennedy, N., Ndoya, N., and Emond, A. (2012). ThermoSpots to detect hypothermia in children with severe acute malnutrition. *PLoS One* 7 (9): e45823.

Motbainor, A., Worku, A., and Kumie, A. (2015). Stunting is associated with food diversity while wasting with food insecurity among under five children in East and West Gojjam Zones of Amhara region, Ethiopia. *PLoS One* 10 (8): e0133542.

Mwangome, M.R., Fegen, G., Fulford, T. et al. (2012). Mid-upper arm circumference at age of routine infant vaccination to identify infants at elevated risk of death: a retrospective cohort study in the Gambia. *Bull. World Health Organ.* 90: 887–894.

Nelson, D.L. and Cox, M.M. (2015). *Lehninger Principles of Biochemistry*, 7e. New York: Macmillan.

Nshimyiryo, A., Hedt-Gauthier, B., Mutaganzwa, C. et al. (2019). Risk factors for stunting among children under five years: a cross-sectional population-based study in Rwanda using the 2015 Demographic and Health Survey. *BMC Public Health* 19: 175.

Pedro, T.M., Kahn, K., Pettifor, J.M. et al. (2014). Under- and overnutrition and evidence of metabolic disease risk in rural black South African children and adolescents. *S. Afr. J. Clin. Nutr.* 27 (4): 198–200.

Pomeroy, E., Stock, J.T., Stanojevic, S. et al. (2014). Stunting, adiposity, and the individual-level 'dual burden' among urban lowland and rural highland Peruvian children. *Am. J. Hum. Biol.* 26: 481–490.

Prado, E.L. and Dewey, K.G. (2014). Nutrition and brain development in early life. *Nutr. Rev.* 72 (4): 267–284.

Prendergast, A.J. and Humphrey, J.H. (2014). The stunting syndrome in developing countries. *Paediatr. Int. Child Health* 34 (4): 250–265.

Puoane, T., Sanders, D., Chopra, M. et al. (2001). Evaluating the clinical management of severely malnourished children – a study of two rural district hospitals. *S. Afr. Med. J.* 91 (2): –137, 141.

Rahman, A., Chowdhury, S., and Hossain, D. (2009). Acute malnutrition in Bangladeshi children: levels and determinants. *Asia Pac. J. Public Health* 21 (3): 294–302.

Rytter, M.J.H., Namusoke, H., Babirekere-Iriso, E. et al. (2015). Social, dietary and clinical correlates of oedema in children with severe acute malnutrition: a cross-sectional study. *BMC Paediatr.* 15 (25).

Schoeman, S., Faber, M., Adams, V. et al. (2010). Adverse social, nutrition and health conditions in rural districts of the KwaZulu Natal and Eastern Cape provinces, South Africa. *South Afr. J. Clin. Nutr.* 23 (3): 140–147.

Shen, Y., Griswold, S., Langlois, B. et al. (2019). Cost and cost-effectiveness of four specialised nutritious foods for treatment of moderate acute malnutrition in Sierra Leone. *Curr. Dev. Nutr.* 3 (S1): 920.

Skolnik, R. (2012). *Global Health 101*, 2e. Burlington, MA: Jones and Bartlett Learning.

Smit, E.N., Muskiet, A.J., and Boersma, E.R. (2004). The possible role of essential fatty acids in the pathophysiology of malnutrition: a review. *Prostaglandins Leukot. Essent. Fatty Acids* 71 (4): 241–250.

Steenkamp, L., Lategan, R., and Raubenheimer, J. (2016). Moderate malnutrition in children aged five years and younger in South Africa: are wasting or stunting being treated? *S. Afr. J. Clin. Nutr.* 29 (1): 27–31.

Stewart, C.P., Ianotti, L.G., Dewey, K.F., and Onyango, A. (2013). Contextualising complementary feeding in a broader framework for stunting prevention. *Matern. Child Nutr.* 9 (S2): 27–45.

Talbert, A., Atkinson, S., Karisa, J. et al. (2009). Hypothermia in children with severe malnutrition: low prevalence on the tropical coast of Kenya. *J. Trop. Paediatr.* 55 (6): 413–416.

Tickell, K.D. and Denno, D.M. (2016). Inpatient management of children with severe acute malnutrition: a review of WHO guidelines. *Bull. World Health Organ.* 94 (9): 642–651.

United Nations Children's Fund (1990). UNICEF Conceptual Framework. https://www.unicef.org/nutrition/training/2.5/4.html (accessed 26 June 2017).

Veldman, F., Kujjura, R., and Kassier, S. (2020). Formulation, sensory attributes and nutrient content of a malted sorghum-based porridge: Potential for the management of moderate acute malnutrition among infants and young children. *Curr. Nutr. Food Sci.* 17 (5): 2021.

Walsh, K., Calder, N., Olupot-Olupot, P. et al. (2018). Modifying intestinal integrity and micro biome in severe malnutrition with legume-based feeds (MIMBLE 2.0): protocol for a phase II refined feed and intervention trial. *Wellcome Open Res.* 3: 95.

Weisstaub, G., Medina, M., Pizarro, F., and Araya, M. (2008). Copper, iron, and zinc status in children with moderate and severe acute malnutrition recovered following WHO protocols. *Biol. Trace Elem. Res.* 124 (1): 1–11.

WHO (2006). *WHO Multicentre Growth Reference Study Group: WHO Child Growth Standards: Length/Height for Age, Weight for Age, Weight for Length, Weight for Height and Body Mass Index for Age: Methods and Development, 2006.* Geneva: World Health Organisation.

WHO (2013). *Guideline: Updates on the Management of Severe Acute Malnutrition in Infants and Children.* Geneva: World Health Organisation.

WHO (2020). Global Health Observatory available from: https://www.who.int/data/gho/data/indicators/indicator-details/GHO/stunting-prevalence accessed on 28 June 2021.

WHO and UNICEF (2009). *WHO Growth Standards and the Identification of Severe Acute Malnutrition in Infants and Children: A Joint Statement by the World Health Organisation and United Nations Children's Fund.* Geneva, Switzerland: World Health Organisation.

World Health Organisation (2011). *Preventing and treating hypothermia in severely malnourished children: Biological, behavioural and contextual rationale.* e-Library of Evidence for Nutrition Actions (eLENA).

World Health Organisation (2017). Media centre: Children: reducing mortality 2017. Available from http://who.int/mediacentre/factsheets/fs178/en accessed on 21/12/2018.

Yebyo, H.G., Kendall, C., Nigusse, D., and Lemma, W. (2013). Outpatient therapeutic feeding program outcomes and determinants in treatment of severe acute malnutrition in Tigray, northern Ethiopia: a retrospective cohort study. *PLoS One* 8 (6): e65840.

Zinc Investigators Collaborative Group (1999). Prevention of diarrhoea and pneumonia by supplementation in children in developing countries: pooled analysis of randomised controlled trials. *J. Paediatr. Dent.* 155: 698–697.

7

Micronutrient Deficiencies – Iron, Iodine, Vitamin A, Zinc and Folate

7.1 Micronutrient Deficiency

Although an individual may be meeting their daily energy requirements, the diet may be deficient in micronutrients. This form of undernutrition does not necessarily result in a feeling of hunger perceived by the individual and is known as 'hidden hunger' (Kennedy et al. 2003). Hidden hunger may be indirectly responsible for poor growth and immune function which may contribute to stunting, underweight and the resulting burden of under-five mortality. In sub-Saharan Africa, it typically includes vitamin A deficiency (VAD) and iron deficiency.

Micronutrient malnutrition describes inadequate or excess intakes of one or more vitamins or minerals. It was known by the sixteenth century that citrus fruits could prevent scurvy in sailors on long voyages. The specific micronutrients responsible for deficiency diseases and disorders first began to be recognised in the late nineteenth and early twentieth centuries. Cell theory led to the discovery of pathogenic organisms, and familiar diseases were investigated by scientists to identify the causative agents. However, all diseases could not be explained by the presence of pathogenic micro-organism exposure. This led to the identification of vitamin B1 (thiamine) deficiency as the cause of beriberi by Christiaan Eijkman, who later won the Nobel prize for his discovery. Deficiency diseases include scurvy, pellagra, beriberi, anaemia, iodine deficiency disorder, xeropthalmia and rickets. All these disease conditions are still recurring challenges in emergency settings today.

Additionally, deficiencies lead to developmental issues including growth retardation and impaired immunity and a consequent increased risk and severity of infectious disease. Nutritional deficiency and infectious disease form part of a cycle, where infectious diseases worsen the problem of an inadequate diet. More than two billion people suffer from some form of micronutrient deficiency worldwide, and this problem leads to poor

Nutrition and Global Health, First Edition. Shawn W. McLaren.
© 2023 John Wiley & Sons Ltd. Published 2023 by John Wiley & Sons Ltd.

child growth and slow economic progress. Vitamin A, zinc, iodine, iron, folate and vitamin B12 requirements are among the most difficult to meet for populations with poor dietary diversity. These are populations that rely on a single staple food for the majority of their caloric requirements.

7.2 Strategies to Address Micronutrient Deficiency

7.2.1 Fortification

Fortification is also known as enrichment. These terms describe the process of adding one or more essential nutrients to a food. It does not matter whether or not the food naturally contains the nutrient being added. The purpose of fortification is to prevent or correct an existing deficiency of specific nutrients in the population or population subgroups (WHO and FAO 2006).

Restoration is another process that is sometimes referred to as enrichment. In this case, essential nutrients that are lost during food processing, storage or handling are added back to the food product. The nutrients are added back in amounts that result in nutrient levels that are the same as those that would be found in the edible portion of the food product before processing, storage or handling (FAO 2003).

Food fortification, restoration or enrichment are medium-term strategies to address micronutrient deficiency. They are also viewed as a supportive strategy to dietary diversification, instead of as an alternative approach, in cases where the existing food supply is limited and is unable to meet the micronutrient requirements of the population. Fortification strategies also require nutrition education and social communication programmes in order to be effective. An advantage of using this strategy is that less change is required for consumer food habits and behaviours. However, it often occurs that fortified foods do not reach consumers in rural areas or target groups located far from central fortification plants. Fortification requires input from stakeholders in government as well as consumers, as policy and regulations are necessary, as well as labelling, quality standards and safety.

Fortification of staple foods on a large scale is considered cost-effective and sustainable as an intervention. This strategy is implemented in both developed and developing countries as a part of public health nutrition policy. The aim of fortification is to promote increased intakes of target nutrients for the majority of the population and to achieve the country's reference nutrient intakes. It is also a method of improving the nutritional status of specific populations or sub-populations, such as women of childbearing age and pregnant women. Fortification of staple foods aims to reduce micronutrient deficiency diseases in populations where intakes are very low.

Food fortification policy needs to consider the intakes of nutrients from unfortified foods and the anticipated consumption of the food to be fortified. Policy also needs to consider the bioavailability of the added nutrients, whether there is a risk of excessive intakes of the fortified nutrients, particularly among consumers who eat an excessive amount of a fortified food, and the likely impact of fortification on overall intake of the nutrient or nutrients.

7.2.1.1 High-Dose Supplementation

VAD is a major health problem in developing regions of the world (WHO 2009). VAD is defined as a serum retinol concentration of less than 7 μmol per litre as per WHO guidelines (WHO 2011), and VAD is related to growth retardation in young children (Castejon et al. 2013).

While food fortification is a medium-term strategy, high-dose supplementation with specific nutrients is often used as a short-term strategy to address micronutrient deficiency. However, in practical terms, high-dose supplementation has become a long-term strategy in some cases, particularly in regions where micronutrient deficiency prevalence is high among vulnerable groups such as pregnant and lactating women and children. Vitamin A capsules are an example of a high-dose supplement, where this strategy has been shown to be rapidly effective. The mortality rate among children aged six months to five years has been reduced through vitamin A supplementation. However, this strategy still requires continuous distribution, supply and investment.

Vitamin A is administered to children younger than five years at six month intervals. These supplements are in the form of oil-based drops containing 100 000–200 00 IU of vitamin A. The WHO recommends a minimum coverage of 80% of the under-five population for vitamin A supplementation to affect child mortality (Sommer et al. 1986). Mayo-Wilson et al. (2011) reported that the provision of high-dose vitamin A capsules resulted in a 24% decrease in all-cause child mortality.

The prevalence of VAD has been slow to respond to the rapid uptake of vitamin A supplementation programmes (Mason et al. 2015); therefore, VAD has not reduced proportionately to the increase in availability of vitamin A supplementation. The criticism for the vitamin A supplementation programme is that the recommendations are 20 years old and have only been tested once (Mason et al. 2015). Mason et al. (2015) report that biannual vitamin A doses do not appear to reduce VAD itself.

Apart from VAD, a report by the WHO/CDC (2008) indicated that globally an estimated 600 million pre-school and school-aged children were anaemic.

Iron supplements are not provided routinely to children in the same manner as vitamin A in the primary healthcare setting. There are concerns that iron supplementation could increase the number of morbidities from infections among children. In a randomised controlled trial, Sazawal et al. (2006) found that supplementation with 12.5 mg iron was related to a higher number of infections in children. A recent randomised, placebo-controlled trial tested the effect of low dose iron supplements (2.5 mg) in the form of a home-based fortification powder (Barth-Jaeggi et al. 2016). Iron supplementation had a significant positive effect on child weight ($P = 0.0038$); however, iron-supplemented participants also reported a higher incidence of coughing ($P = 0.003$) and dyspnoea ($P = 0.0002$) than those receiving the placebo (Barth-Jaeggi et al. 2016). It was also found that supplementation was not effective in improving iron status. It is possible that doses of iron were too low and that a high prevalence of helminth infestations and infections rendered the supplemented iron ineffective (Barth-Jaeggi et al. 2016).

In a systematic review of randomised controlled trials, Sachdev et al. (2006) found that iron supplementation had no significant effect on the growth of children. The iron supplementation interventions reviewed included oral and parenteral iron supplements as well as iron-fortified infant formula and infant cereals. None of these interventions had any significant effect on the weight for age (WFA), weight for height (WFH), height for age (HFA) or mid-upper arm circumference (MUAC) of infants and young children (Sachdev et al. 2006). Although iron deficiency thus appears to affect growth, it is uncertain whether prophylactic use of iron supplements may prevent malnutrition.

7.2.1.2 Childhood Anaemia

Childhood anaemia is common and causes developmental delays. Children younger than two years of age are at a higher risk of anaemia. Children with anaemic mothers are more likely to be anaemic themselves. Low levels of maternal education and low household income are also linked to a higher likelihood of children being anaemic. Poor sanitation is an important determinant of poor iron status.

Anaemia in children can be caused by nutritional deficit in iron intake and is associated with other forms of malnutrition. It may be the result of infection. In some children, anaemia is caused by genetic disorders and haemoglobinopathies such as sickle cell anaemia or thalassaemia. Anaemia can also be associated with chronic diseases.

Haemoglobin levels (g/dl) for diagnosis of anaemia in children (WHO 2011)

Age	Non-anaemic	Anaemia		
		Mild	Moderate	Severe
6 months to 5 years	>11.0	10.0–10.9	7.0–9.9	<7.0
5–11 years	>11.5	11.0–11.5	8.0–10.9	<8.0
12–14 years	>12.0	11.0–11.9	8.0–10.9	<8.0

Iron is required for the synthesis of haem. Transferring iron saturation is an indicator of iron stores in the body. When body stores of iron are adequate, the protein hepcidin is produced, which reduces absorption of iron from the gastrointestinal tract. However, iron absorption may be affected by external factors. Non-haem iron is less readily absorbed. Common staple foods such as maize, millet, rice and beans contain low concentrations of haem-iron. Common staples also contain inhibitory factors including phytates and tannins which reduce the body's ability to absorb iron. Iron absorption is inhibited by phytic acid and non-starch polysaccharides in foods. These compounds are predominantly found in the bran from cereal grains. Ascorbic acid partly counteracts this inhibition (Minihane and Rimbach 2002).

Among children in low- and middle-income countries, anaemia has been associated with maternal anaemia. Household wealth, maternal education and low birthweight are also factors associated with childhood anaemia (Prieto-Petron et al. 2018). Children who consume fortified foods, potatoes and other tubers have lower rates of anaemia (Prieto-Petron et al. 2018).

Important nutrition-sensitive interventions to prevent childhood anaemia include improvements in education for women, reducing poverty, delayed childbearing and wider birth spacing through the provision of adequate family planning services (Prieto-Petron et al. 2018). Nutrition-specific interventions include the introduction of iron-rich foods during the complementary feeding stage after six months of age.

7.2.2 Adult Anaemia

7.2.2.1 Iron Deficiency Anaemia

Iron deficiency anaemia is one of the most common forms of malnutrition among adults across the world and is particularly problematic among women of childbearing age. It occurs in approximately 2–5% of men and post-menopausal women. Among men and post-menopausal women, gastrointestinal blood loss is the most common cause of iron deficiency anaemia (Goddard et al. 2011). Menstrual blood loss is the most common cause of iron deficiency anaemia among premenopausal women. It occurs when iron absorption from the diet is insufficient to cover iron losses. Causes include poor iron intake, high iron losses or increased physiological demands for iron which are not matched by increased dietary intake of iron.

Factors associated with anaemia in sub-Saharan Africa include exposure to malaria and HIV. Pregnant women are at a higher risk of anaemia in this region. Younger women, between the ages of 25 and 35 years, who are poorly educated, have a low income and live in urban areas are also at a higher risk of anaemia (Correa-Agudela et al. 2021).

Iron deficiency anaemia is commonly diagnosed when features such as fatigue, pica, nail changes or hair loss occur. The term pica refers to the practice of regularly consuming non-food items. Commonly consumed items may include frost, ice, raw starched, stones and sand (Roy et al. 2018). The practice has been associated with low iron stores as well as food insecurity among pregnant women (Roy et al. 2018).

VAD may exacerbate the problem of anaemia. Vitamin A is involved in iron homeostasis, immune function, erythropoietin expression and apoptosis of erythrocyte precursors.

Anaemia is defined as:

- haemoglobin <130 g/l (13 g/dl) in men older than age 15 years,
- haemoglobin <120 g/l (12 g/dl) in non-pregnant women older than age 15 years and
- haemoglobin <110 g/l (11 g/dl) in pregnant women (World Health Organisation 2008).

7.2.2.2 Treatment for Anaemia

Iron deficiency anaemia may be treated with supplementation using iron tablets. The use of iron supplementation to alleviate iron-deficiency anaemia requires a strong supply, distribution and availability of the tablets. It is important to note that the tablets may deteriorate if stored over very long periods of time. It is also very important to note that iron supplementation will only treat anaemia when the cause of anaemia is iron deficiency. In cases where anaemia is due to another aetiology, patients will not respond to iron supplementation. It is recommended that patients should be treated with anti-malarial medications, anti-helminth chemotherapy, antibiotics and folate supplements as required.

Severe anaemia requires more intensive treatment, particularly if it is complicated by shock, heart failure or dehydration. The WHO recommends that the transfusions of haemoglobin should be lower than 4 g/dl.

7.3 Iodine

Iodine deficiency disorders are the most common cause of cognitive developmental delay in the world. Iodine deficiency results in goitre, poor cognitive function (Lazarus 2015) and hyper and hypothyroidism. Severe iodine deficiency during pregnancy results in cretinism. Iodine content of food is largely determined by the iodine concentration in the soil it is grown in, with some mountainous or river-bed settlements such as those in the Andes and along the Ganges river having a high risk for iodine deficiency. Globalisation and worldwide food distribution and the uptake of iodised salt have resulted in reduced rates of cretinism.

7.3.1 Role of Iodine in Human Health

Iodine is an integral part of thyroid hormones. Thyroid hormones regulate body temperature. They are also important for cell reproduction, growth and blood cell production, and play roles in nerve and muscle function. Importantly, thyroid hormones control the rate of oxygen consumption by cells and therefore affect the basal metabolic rate and metabolism.

7.3.2 Thyroid Physiology

Thyroid hormone production is regulated by the hypothalamus, which controls the release of thyroid stimulating hormone (TSH). TSH acts on the thyroid and causes the thyroid gland to release thyroxine, one of the thyroid hormones. Thyroxine is also known as tetraiodothyronine (T4). Once T4 reaches target cells, it loses one iodine and becomes triiodothyronine (T3), the active form of the thyroid hormone (Figure 7.1).

Na$^+$ K$^+$ ATPase pumps play a role in basal metabolism. Cells expend large amounts of energy to maintain the correct concentration gradients of Na$^+$, K$^+$, H$^+$ and Ca^{2+} across the plasma and intracellular membranes (Lodish et al. 2000). Up to 25% of ATP in nerve and kidney cells is expended for ion transport, and up to 50% of ATP in erythrocytes is used for this purpose. Na$^+$ K$^+$ ATPase pumps are activated by T3.

Genetically obese mice show lower oxygen consumption and greater efficiency of energy utilization than their littermates. Muscle membranes from obese mice have fewer ouabain binding sites per milligram of protein, but there is no difference in binding affinity. This lower sodium pump (Na+, K+ – ATPase) activity suggests a mechanism for decreased thermogenesis in obese mice

Thyroid physiology

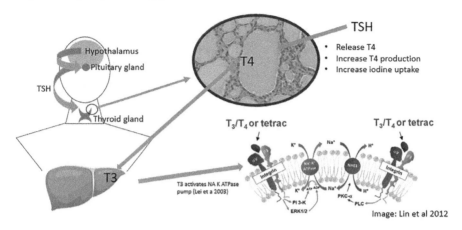

Figure 7.1: Thyroid physiology and the role of thyroid hormones in basal metabolism.

Source: Adapted from Lei et al. 2003.

7.3.3 Iodine Deficiency

Iodine deficiency results in reduced thyroid hormone production. The hypothalamus responds by producing more TSH to increase iodine uptake. Iodine deficiency causes the thyroid gland to swell, in order to catch as much iodine as possible, which results in goitre. Goitre is a visible enlargement of the thyroid gland. When goitre is caused by iodine deficiency in this manner, it is known as simple goitre. Almost all cases of goitre are simple goitre.

Iodine deficiency is a cause of mental impairment and brain damage (Bernal 2005) and is the most common cause of mental impairment worldwide. Mild deficiency in iodine results in poor school performance in children.

7.3.4 Iodine Deficiency Disorders Through the Life Cycle

Iodine is required for normal development of the foetal nervous system (Figure 7.2). Severe iodine deficiency during pregnancy causes cretinism in children, characterised by extreme and irreversible mental and physical stunting. This is because iodine deficiency results in reduced thyroid hormone production (hypothyroxinaemia) in the pregnant mother. Thyroxine is important for brain development in the foetus. During the first and second trimesters, the majority of the foetal thyroid hormones are made by the mother and reach the developing foetus via the placenta (De Escobar et al. 2004). Hypothyroxinaemia in early pregnancy results

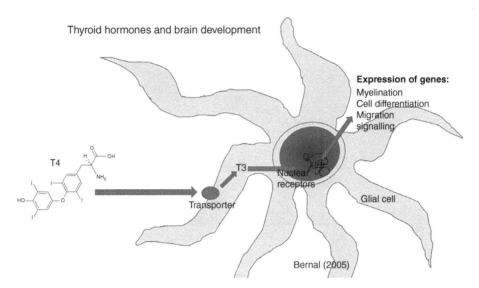

Thyroid hormones and brain development

Figure 7.2: The role of thyroid hormones in brain development.
Source: Adapted from Bernal (2005).

in endemic cretinism, and in later pregnancy it results in severe thyroid insufficiency, stunted growth, delayed sexual development and a lesser degree of neurologic impairment and mental deficiency (Eastman and Zimmerman 2000).

Neonates with iodine deficiency are born with elevated levels of TSH. They have an increased risk of perinatal mortality and higher rates of congenital abnormalities. It is also more likely that they will be born with a low birthweight.

Childhood iodine deficiency results in goitre and may cause subclinical hypothyroidism or hyperthyroidism. It causes impaired mental function and physical development.

There are higher rates of apathy among adults in iodine-deficient areas as iodine deficiency affects initiative and decision-making abilities. Adults who are deficient in iodine can develop symptoms including goitre with complications, impaired mental function and hypothyroidism. Iodine deficiency can cause spontaneous hyperthyroidism in adults and can result in increased susceptibility of the thyroid gland to nuclear radiation.

7.3.5 Causes of Iodine Deficiency Disorders

Iodine deficiency disorders are related to the quality of the soil in which crops are grown. Soil with low iodine concentrations results in poor iodine uptake by crops (Figure 7.3). This is particularly common in mountainous regions and regions prone to flooding such as the Ganges river and Andes (De Benoist et al. 2004).

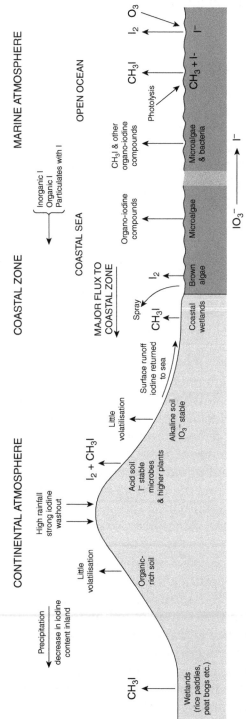

Figure 7.3: Geographical factors affecting availability of iodine.

Goitrogens are found in legumes, cruciferous vegetables – cabbage, cauliflower, broccoli, turnip and forms of root cassava.

Soy- or soy-enriched foods can also aggravate thyroid problems reducing T4 absorption and interfering with thyroid hormone action (Bajaj et al. 2016).

7.3.6 Excess Dietary Iodine

In genetically susceptible individuals, increased consumption of iodine can cause thyroiditis. Foods high in iodine include kelp, seaweed, iodinated salt, iodine additives to bread and flour, preservatives, medicines such as amiodarone and vitamin supplements. The foetus can develop goitre in utero when exposed to excess iodine. It is thought that excessive iodine exposure has a toxic effect on the thyroid gland through the action of oxygen free radicals and over-stimulation of the immune system.

7.3.7 Strategies to Address Iodine Deficiency

Iodine fortification was pioneered in Switzerland in 1922. Now table salt, livestock feed and staple foods such as bread and dairy products are fortified with iodine (Fuge and Johnson 2015). This is thought to be a cost-effective intervention due to the low cost of fortification.

The natural history of iodine deficiency disorders across populations in areas with high prevalence is initially counter-intuitive when iodine fortification is introduced. Severe iodine deficiency results in goitre and hypothyroidism. This is because there is insufficient iodine available to allow for normal production of thyroid hormone. In individuals from iodine-deficient populations with mild to moderate iodine deficiency, the thyroid gland compensates for iodine deficiency by increasing its activity and therefore maintains euthyroidism. However, chronic thyroid over-stimulation increases hyperthyroidism risk and toxic nodular goitre prevalence in these populations (Zimmerman and Boelaert 2015).

There is a further increase in hyperthyroidism prevalence if iodine intake is increased significantly by salt iodisation. This is the part that is initially counter-intuitive; however, it makes sense under closer inspection in the context of iodine toxicity. Furthermore, the increase in prevalence is transient as iodine sufficiency normalises thyroid activity and reduces nodular autonomy. It should be noted that increased iodine intake in an iodine-deficient population is associated with a small increase in the prevalence of subclinical hypothyroidism and thyroid autoimmunity; whether these increases are also transient is unclear.

Methods of improving iodine status include iodisation and supplementation. Iodisation of commonly consumed foods is a longer-term solution, whereas supplementation is a short-term solution used until iodised salt becomes universal. Iodisation is a strategy employed on entire populations, whereas supplementation is targeted at iodine deficiency endemic areas. Salt is widely used as a food product for iodisation. Levels of goitre have improved in Italy since the introduction of iodised salt in 2005. Tea is fortified with iodine in Tibet, bread in Holland and Australia, and drinking water in Thailand and Italy. Iodine supplementation is administered in the form of iodine oil, injections or capsules. They are administered every five years, targeting women and children in endemic regions.

7.4 Vitamin A Deficiency

VAD is a preventable cause of blindness and is important for immune system function and normal growth and development. Millions of children and women of childbearing age are vitamin A-deficient worldwide. Treatment and prevention strategies include vitamin A supplementation, food fortification and community gardening.

7.4.1 Vitamin A Forms and Food Sources

There are two forms of compounds that can function as vitamin A. The first is preformed vitamin A, and this group is made up of retinol, retinal and retinoic acid. The second form is the provitamin A carotenoids. There are at least 50 carotenoids that can be converted to vitamin A. Carotenoids are converted to retinal or retinoic acid in the liver or intestinal cells. Retinol is found in animal products including eggs, liver and dairy foods. Provitamin A carotenoids are found in plants, and dietary sources of these compounds include green leafy vegetables, orange or yellow fruits and vegetables, and red palm oil.

Around 80% of the vitamin A in African diets comes from carotenoids in plant foods such as spinach, amaranth, cow pea leaves and sweet potato. Other sources of preformed retinol are mainly derived from milk and eggs (Codija 2001).

7.4.2 Vitamin A Functions

Vitamin A is a fat-soluble vitamin with a range of roles which include promoting vision, cell differentiation, immune system function, promoting growth and bone remodelling. Vitamin A plays a vital role in cell differentiation. Retinoic acid influences the production, structure and function of epithelial cells both externally and internally. It is also involved in erythropoiesis – the formation of new red blood cells. As vitamin A plays an important role in cell differentiation, it supports immune function. Vitamin A maintains the mucous membranes in the gastrointestinal tract and respiratory tract. When there is VAD, the function of these membranes is impaired.

7.4.3 Consequences of Vitamin A Deficiency

VAD is a public health problem in 118 countries, particularly affecting the African and Southeast Asian regions. Approximately 100–140 million children are vitamin A deficient across the world and are the most important cause of preventable blindness in children in low- and middle-income countries.

VAD causes nyctalopia or night blindness, which is an early sign of functional deterioration. When vitamin A depletion progresses further to severe states, the result is dry eyes, keratomalacia and blindness.

VAD results in reduced resistance to infection, and a consequent increased risk of severe illness and death from common infections. These include measles and diarrheal diseases. Approximately 60% of children with VAD presenting with xeropthalmia die within one year due to infectious disease.

As vitamin A plays an important role in cell differentiation, all body surfaces internally and externally are affected by VAD. Skin becomes coarse and thickened, and the lining of the mouth and gastrointestinal tract and lungs are damaged. VAD causes growth failure in children and is a common cause of stunting. When the gut mucosa is damaged or not functioning correctly, this leads to poor absorption of nutrients. This common problem responds well to supplementation with vitamin A, and supplementation corresponds with weight gain and improved growth rates.

7.4.4 Causes of Vitamin A Deficiency

VAD is caused by poor intake and can be exacerbated by increased requirements for vitamin A or poor absorption. Diets in low- and middle-income countries are based on starchy staple foods with less contribution from fat, dairy products, fruits and vegetables.

VAD is linked with socio-economic factors and is often found in the same population sub-groups as iron deficiency anaemia, including infants and young children and women of reproductive age. Physiological requirements for vitamin A are increased during pregnancy and are high during childhood and periods of illness.

7.4.5 Prevention of Vitamin A Deficiency

The most effective preventive policy for VAD is implementing the use of high-dose supplements. Many countries have policies for routine supplementation for women and children.

Population group	Oral dose	Frequency of dose
Infants 0–6 months	50000 IU	Once
Infants 6–12 months	100000 IU	Every 4–6 months
Children >1 year	200000 IU	Every 4–6 months
Pregnant and other fertile women	Not more than 10000 IU	Daily
Breastfeeding women	200000 IU	Once during the first 8 weeks after delivery

7.4.6 Vitamin A Supplementation Programmes

Vitamin A supplementation programmes are often linked with wider nutrition programmes and immunisation programmes. For example, vitamin A supplementation is often incorporated into Expanded Programme for Immunisation (EPI) planning as children can then receive both treatments simultaneously. Bangladesh makes use of biannual micronutrient days to provide vitamin A supplementation coverage. Vitamin A has been incorporated into multiple micronutrient supplementations for women of childbearing age.

However, progress is slow in improving coverage of vitamin A supplementation and this has impacted the effectiveness of the programmes and associated mortality reduction. The results of studies on the effectiveness of vitamin A supplementation to reduce childhood morbidity and mortality have been inconsistent (Gebremedhin 2017). The supplements themselves are a cost-effective intervention, but the main cost is in the delivery system. In spite of challenges to implementing the vitamin A supplementation programme, many countries are using vitamin A supplementation as a method to reduce diarrhoeal disease in children.

Another effective strategy is to use food-based approaches. Commonly consumed foods such as sugar, cereals, flours, margarine and oils are fortified with vitamin A. Instant noodles are fortified with vitamin A in southeast Asia, and Guatemala fortifies its sugar. Vegetable oil may be fortified with vitamin A, and recently most major donors and the World Food Programme have made it policy that vegetable oils are fortified with vitamin A. World Food programme specifications are that vegetable oil must be fortified with vitamin A at 24 000–36 000 IU/kg. As vitamin A is light sensitive, fortified oils should be stored in light-proof containers.

Rice is a staple food for more than 3 billion people. In South Asia, rice can contribute as much as two-thirds of the daily caloric intake. While milled rice is a good source of energy, it is a poor source of micronutrients. Rice has therefore been proposed as a good candidate for fortification. However, fortification of rice has been slowed due to technical problems, with some effective interventions based on more recent technological advances. As fortification of rice has proven challenging, complementary biofortification and dietary diversification need to be considered as important strategies.

People with access to small homestead or community gardens are encouraged to grow vitamin A-rich foods in order to promote dietary diversification and improve vitamin A intake. This can be enhanced with small animal production, such as keeping chickens for eggs. Fermentation and malting grown produce have also been shown to improve micronutrient status. Enhancing small homestead or community agriculture is a long-term strategy. It increases the quantity of micronutrient-rich foods consumed though improved access and availability. Community gardens have been shown to significantly increase the amount of vitamin A consumed by children (Faber et al. 2002). An interesting outcome of homestead agriculture projects has been that vitamin A consumption improves even among children from homes without vegetable gardens. This is a result of parents bargaining for neighbours' produce, sharing produce or selling produce such as butternut squash to local shops (Faber et al. 2002).

Challenges to implementing community vegetable gardens include lack of fencing, animals eating crops and a lack of water (Zimpita et al. 2015). Overcoming these challenges yields significant and sustainable results for vegetable and fruit consumption and micronutrient status. Evidence suggests that even three years after a vegetable gardening intervention in a community, crop yields are sustained, with as much as 43 kg of produce per household per year (Baliki et al. 2019). Alongside improved access to micronutrient-dense food, long-term outcomes of community vegetable gardening include improvements in women's nutrition knowledge and behavioural change (Baliki et al. 2019). Vegetable gardens can also have an impact on women's empowerment as they encourage market participation even when programmes are only modest in scope (Baliki et al. 2019).

7.4.7 Strategies for Addressing Iron and VAD

Strategies for addressing iron and VAD may focus on increasing production, increasing uptake or increasing bioavailability of these two nutrients. By increasing the production of iron- and vitamin A-rich foods, the availability of these nutrients will be improved. This may be achieved by encouraging home production of foods high in vitamin A and iron. Increasing the consumption of these iron- and vitamin A-rich foods may be improved through nutrition education. This may be achieved through social marketing and behaviour change strategies, which increase the social desirability and emphasise the nutritional value of these foods for improving diet quality. Bioavailability may be improved through home preservation and processing techniques. The mnemonic 'SLAMENGHI' (West and Castenmiller 1998) is sometimes used to remember the aspects of foods that can be adjusted to affect bioavailability:

- (S) species of vegetable or compound of interest;
- (L) molecular linkage;
- (A) amount of carotenoids consumed;
- (M) matrix;
- (E) effectors of absorption and bioconversion
- (N) nutrient status of host;
- (G) genetic factors;
- (H) host-related factors;
- (I) interactions.

Carotene-rich foods given to VAD patients with low liver and plasma vitamin A concentrations have been shown to elevate vitamin A plasma levels. In some studies, the addition of fat has been shown to significantly increase plasma vitamin A levels.

In addition, plant breeding strategies such as producing golden rice and yellow maize should be included with the benefits involved in GM technology to alleviate micronutrient deficiencies.

According to De Groote et al. (2010), there are three major public health strategies for addressing the issue of VAD in sub-Saharan Africa. The first approach is industrial fortification. Industrial fortification is a form of exogenous fortification (Nuss and Tanumihardjo 2016). This is the practice of adding micronutrients to other food products during processing or packaging (De Groot et al. 2010). Typically, a multivitamin premix may be added to staple flour (Nuss and Tanumihardjo 2016). The second approach has been to create awareness of the VAD problem in affected areas. This strategy relies on public nutrition education on the importance of dietary diversity (De Groote et al. 2010). This aims to address the underlying cause of VAD as defined by the WHO (2009).

The third approach is to provide children with vitamin A supplements every six months. This is a very popular strategy in developing countries (De Groote et al. 2010). This approach to addressing the VAD problem has also been considered as a very cost-effective measure (IVACG 2003).

These strategies have shown some level of success in the South African context. According to SANHANES-1 (2013), the national prevalence of VAD in children under five has decreased by 20% since the first national nutritional surveys conducted post-1994. This may be due to the successes of the vitamin A supplementation programme affecting this age group. However, limitations hinder further success in other sections of the population.

In spite of the successes seen due to supplementation, this strategy is still limited in rural areas with poor transport infrastructure (De Groote et al. 2010). People in rural areas have poorer access to healthcare systems, which inhibit routine supplementation (Mayer et al. 2008).

Mayer et al. (2008) also describe poverty as a barrier to success for food diversification. Thus, a lack of purchasing power prevents information on the importance of dietary diversity from being a practical solution.

According to De Groote et al. (2010), industrial fortification is only a feasible strategy if it involves food products that are consumed widely. As sub-Saharan Africa is still a developing region, the majority of people still live in rural settings. A large proportion of the population's food is processed within the homestead. According to Mayer et al. (2008), a lack of purchasing power and inadequate access to markets are responsible for this. Thus, industrially fortified foods fail to improve the vitamin A status of very large numbers of people. As these strategies have thus far failed to alleviate the VAD problem, new approaches are being developed; biofortification of crops is one of the strategies being currently tried.

7.4.7.1 Biofortification as a Strategy to Combat VAD

One of the approaches being investigated as a means to reduce the prevalence of VAD is known as biofortification. Biofortification aims to improve the nutritional qualities of food crops. It is a form of endogenous fortification (Nuss and Tanumihardjo 2016) in that the crops themselves are adapted to contain higher intrinsic levels of specific nutrients. This is performed through methods of conventional breeding or genetic modification (Nuss and Tanumihardjo 2016). Several of the world's staple crops have been targeted for biofortification. These include rice, wheat, beans, cassava, maize and sweet potato (Mayer et al. 2008).

Sweet potatoes biofortified with provitamin A have already shown some potential successes (De Groote et al. 2010). This has been quantified by observed increases in vitamin A intake and serum retinol concentrations among young children (De Groote et al. 2010). Rice that has been biofortified with provitamin A, known as golden rice, has been developed to contain higher concentrations of provitamin A B-carotenes. This is because polished rice, as it is traditionally consumed as a staple, is typically very low in provitamin A components (Mayer et al. 2008).

7.5 Zinc Deficiency

Zinc is involved in over 200 enzymatic reactions and plays a role in immune function. Deficiency of this mineral results in growth retardation and failure to thrive, diarrhoea, immune suppression, skin and eye lesions. There is growing evidence that mild zinc deficiency is widespread.

7.5.1 The Role of Zinc in Human Physiology

Zinc is an important micronutrient which is involved in nutrient metabolism, collagen formation, sexual maturation, cell replication and growth among other roles in human physiology. Zinc forms part of co-enzymes in a wide range of reactions taking place in the body, including DNA–RNA polymerase; superoxide dismutase, an antioxidant that helps protect the body against reactive oxygen species; alkaline phosphatase (ALP), an important liver enzyme involved in protein catabolism; and carbolic anhydrase, an enzyme found in red blood cells.

7.5.2 Consequences of Zinc Deficiency

Zinc deficiency results in poor wound healing, suboptimal growth, abnormal taste and smell, and impaired reproductive system development. Systemic symptoms of zinc deficiency include growth retardation, immune dysfunction and infection.

7.5.3 Prevalence of Zinc Deficiency

Approximately one third of the global population is deficient in zinc (Caulfield and Black 2004). The prevalence of zinc deficiency in Ethiopia is estimated to be between 51.9% and 67.7% of the population, with 28.4 to 49.4% of pregnant women and children deficient in zinc (Berhe et al. 2019). Low intakes of animal source foods and poor dietary diversity are associated with inadequate zinc status (Berhe et al. 2019). In India, poor intakes of absorbable zinc affects a large segment of the population, with an increase in inadequate intake from 17.1% in 1983 to 24.6% in 2012 (Smith et al. 2019). This corresponds to an additional 82 million people at risk of deficiency (Smith et al. 2019).

7.5.3.1 Strategies to Address Zinc Deficiency

Assessing zinc status presents many challenges as there is still much to be understood about the bioavailability, storage and homeostatic regulation of zinc status (Young et al. 2014). Subclinical zinc deficiency cannot be identified through testing serum zinc levels. Storage of zinc in the human body is depleted quickly by gastrointestinal illness. Therefore, acute gastrointestinal illness is a cause of zinc depletion and deficiency. Deficiency resulting from diarrhoea appears to respond well to supplementation with zinc. Zinc supplementation is used as a treatment for diarrhoea and is recommended by the WHO and UNICEF for use in cases of diarrhoea related to acute malnutrition. It is not well understood why zinc supplementation in children younger than 12 months is less effective (Young et al. 2014).

Strategies for addressing zinc deficiency include maintaining zinc repletion through regular supplementation as a method of preventing deficiency of this nutrient. Secondary prevention takes place during bouts of acute diarrhoea. Further research is needed on the method for administering zinc as a primary preventative (public health) strategy for preventing zinc deficiency. Research needs to address the bioavailability of zinc in various formulations (Young et al. 2014).

7.5.4 Folate

7.5.4.1 Functions of Folate

Folate is made up of a ring structure attached to glutamate. Naturally occurring folate has a polyglutamate structure – up to six glutamate molecules are attached to the basic ring structure. The synthetic form of this vitamin, folic acid, has a monoglutamate structure – only one glutamate molecule is attached. Folic acid is easier to absorb as the additional glutamate on folate must be cleaved off before absorption (Figure 7.4). Folate, together with cobalamin, is involved in nucleic acid production. As it plays a crucial role in nucleic acid production, folate is particularly important for cells with a high turnover rate, such as red blood cells, which have an average life span of approximately three months. Folate

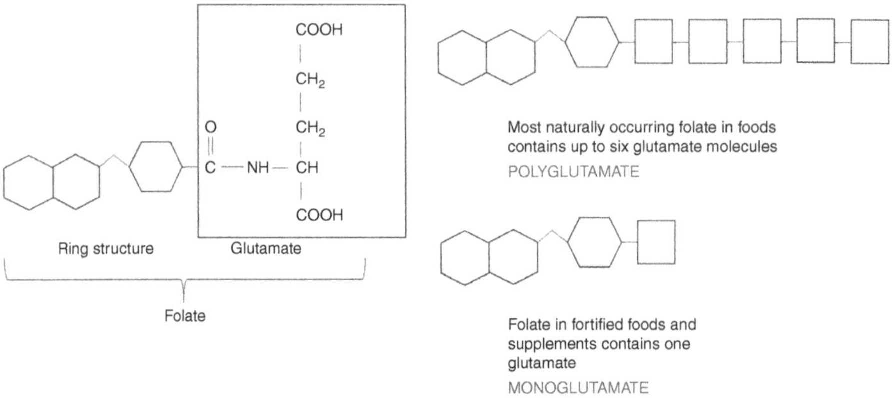

Figure 7.4: Folate structure and absorption.

coenzymes within the cell are involved in one-carbon transfer reactions, including those involved in phases of amino acid metabolism, histidine metabolism and purine and pyrimidine synthesis.

Deficiency of folate results in anaemia, glossitis, neurological disturbances and elevated homocysteine. Folate deficiency results in anaemia because the precursors to nucleic acids required for new cells cannot be produced. Cells with high turnover rates such as the erythrocytes, of which approximately 3 million cells are produced and 3 million are recycled every day, are affected. Elevated folate levels can mask vitamin B12 deficiency. Folate deficiency can therefore also result in poor growth among children. Folate status is particularly important in early pregnancy. While the mechanism is unclear, it is known that folate fortification results in lower rates of neural tube defects in newborns. These neural tube defects include spina bifida and anencephaly. Spina bifida presents with an exposed spinal cord that has not completely closed. In normal foetal development, the spinal cord closes at around 21 days after conception, during the embryonic phase. As this takes place very early into gestation, many women may not yet be aware that they are pregnant before the effect has taken place. Evidence from the Dutch famine showed that rates of neural tube defects increased among infants born to women who conceived during the famine. Rates of neural tube defects decreased among women who conceived approximately three months after the end of the famine. This has informed advice around folic acid supplementation and mandatory folic acid fortification as strategies to prevent neural tube defects. There is a high prevalence of marginal folate deficiency among women of childbearing age.

7.5.5 Strategies to Address Folate Deficiency

Food-first approaches include nutrition education centred around foods that are high in folate. Good food sources of folate include legumes, vegetables and fortified grain products. Rich sources of folate include liver, green leafy vegetables such as spinach and brussels sprouts, okra, legumes and orange juice. Approximately 50% of folate is lost from foods during food processing and cooking. Ascorbic acid acts as a reducing agent and can help protect folate from degradation.

Other approaches include supplementation and fortification. Supplementation is recommended during pregnancy as folate requirements increase during this stage of the life cycle. Requirements increase by approximately 0.4 mg per day during pregnancy. This additional folic acid is needed by the foetus, as well as for producing new tissues, including producing new red blood cells (although haemodilution masks the increase in the number of red blood cells during pregnancy). It is recommended that women of childbearing age supplement with folic acid for at least one month prior to conception to ensure repletion of this nutrient during the early stages of gestation. A supplement of 5 mg per day is recommended for women with a previous history of neural tube defect infants, obesity and type 2 diabetes until the 12th week of pregnancy.

Mandatory fortification with folic acid has been employed as a public health strategy to prevent folate deficiency and neural tube defects in many countries around the world. Following decades of debate and consultation, mandatory fortification of flour with folic acid was approved in the United Kingdom in 2021. Mandatory fortification of staple foods is a safe intervention as the greatest increases in folate status are seen among people with inadequate folate intakes, while the level of fortification is low enough to ensure that people with already adequate intakes do not exceed the upper limit recommendations. Mandatory fortification of flour products with folic acid has been shown to reduce the rates of neural tube defects by up to 25%.

7.6 Conducting a Systematic Search

Nutrition is an evidence-based practice (EBP), which draws on the literature to inform best practice. This section provides information on how to use online databases of studies to perform a literature search, using the effectiveness of vitamin A supplementation as a worked example.

7.6.1 The Purpose of Evidence-Based Practice

EBP is the integration of the best research practice, clinical expertise and patients' values and circumstances.

The term evidence-based medicine was first developed in the field of medicine in the early 1990s, but as its use expanded to include other health disciplines, it became known as EBP. EBP provides a framework for the integration of research evidence and patients' values and preferences into the delivery of healthcare.

7.6.2 Considerations for Evidence-Based Practice

Valid information is needed daily to inform decision-making. Diagnostic skills and clinical judgement improve over time with experience, whereas up-to-date knowledge and clinical performance decline with age and experience. Clinicians lack the time to find and assimilate evidence. Gaps exist between evidence and practice which results in suboptimal practice and quality of care. There is a potential discordance between a pathophysiological and empirical approach to thinking about whether or not something is effective.

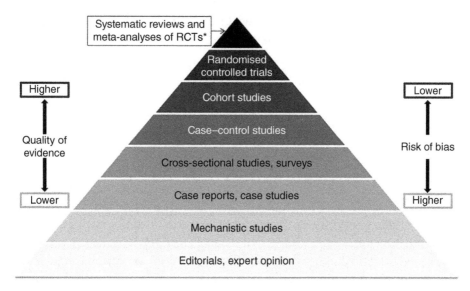

Figure 7.5: Hierarchy of scientific evidence according to study design – as the risk of bias decreases, the quality of the evidence increases.

It is very useful for health workers to be able to identify the preferred study designs for each type of clinical question, as well as the risks and benefits of the main study designs. This requires health workers to be able to classify the main study designs for each type of clinical question. It is also useful to be able to differentiate using research to inform clinical decision-making and conducting research (Albarqouni et al. 2018).

7.6.2.1 Sources of Information

Sources of research information include biomedical research databases. Filtered and pre-appraised evidence sources exist to help clinicians and health workers. The advantages of using filtered and pre-appraised evidence sources are that a fuller breadth of the available evidence can be found in one place, and the conclusions that can be drawn from these sources provide insights that are not possible when looking at the individual papers. The hierarchy of evidence ranks types of studies based on their strength of evidence, contrasted with the risk of bias (Figure 7.5). Well-designed studies reduce the risk of bias as much as possible.

7.6.2.2 Search Strategy

A general search strategy includes search terms, inclusion and exclusion criteria. Searches can be improved using Boolean operators, truncation and by applying search filters. These tools help to improve the efficiency of searches. The search terms used should be built from the research question or PICO method. This will yield a focused and well-defined search that is more likely to answer the research question.

7.6.3 Conducting a Search Using Boolean Operators

PubMed's advanced search allows users to build Boolean search operators. The advantage of this tool is that it allows researchers to look up the types of studies they are looking for more efficiently. If we wanted to evaluate the evidence for vitamin A supplementation during pregnancy, we could build a search strategy to search for this topic specifically. One problem that Boolean operators help to address is the variation in terms used in publications for the same concept. For example, when searching for 'vitamin A' only, the database will not return papers that discuss 'retinol' or 'retinoic acid', even though these other terms will also be relevant. 'Vitamin A' and 'retinol' can be linked as alternative terms using an 'OR' function. We would like to find papers that use vitamin A supplementation for the population group we are interested in and can link the two concepts with an 'AND' function. Similarly, we can incorporate the outcomes we are interested in using the 'AND' function. Boolean operators also include the 'NOT' function, which will exclude papers containing terms we do not wish to include. This can be used to narrow the search to only papers dealing with a particular outcome – for example maternal morbidity, and not low birthweight infants as an outcome – or to eliminate ambiguous terms. Once we have applied these steps, we can generate a search term that might look something like this:

$$\left(\frac{\left(\left(\left(\left(\text{vitamin A}\right)\text{OR}\left(\text{retinol}\right)\right)\text{AND}\left(\text{maternal}\right)\right)\text{AND}\left(\text{pregnancy}\right)\right)}{\text{AND}\left(\text{maternal mortality}\right)\text{AND}\left(\text{supplementation}\right)} \right)$$

7.6.4 Evaluating Evidence – and Tools for Evaluating Evidence

Appraising the integrity, reliability and applicability of health-based research is valuable when interpreting the available evidence. There are tools available online, which enable researchers and practitioners to critically appraise evidence in a systematic way. These tools include the checklists developed by the Critical Appraisal Skills Programme (CASP), the Cochrane Risk of Bias tools, as well as more specialised checklists aimed at particular study designs such as the QUADAS2 tool. Bias in studies may be present in many forms, but it generally stems from the sample selection, the statistical analyses performed or publication of results. Health workers should also be able to recognise the main forms of bias in studies and the way that these biases will affect the interpretation of the results. Having some understanding of the statistics presented in a scientific article can enrich the interpretation of results of the study. Health workers should be aware of the difference between random error and systematic error as sources of bias (Grellety and Golden 2016). Confidence intervals are frequently used to represent the likelihood that the true measure of a phenomenon is where it has been reported. A 95% confidence interval is calculated with an alpha level of 0.05. A wide confidence interval represents more uncertainty in the true location of the result than a smaller confidence interval. When it comes to interpreting odds ratios, a 95% confidence interval which does not cross 0 can be considered statistically significant. As an example, a 95% confidence interval of -0.23 to -0.02 does not cross 0 and can be considered statistically significant. A 95% confidence interval that crosses 0 is not statistically significant and it could be interpreted that we are confident that the effect of the treatment both increases and decreases the measure of effect. It is also worth noting that association does not imply causation. It is important to recognise the importance of conflict of interest and funding sources when reading scientific articles. Authors are usually required to declare any interests that they have when submitting a paper for publication, and this declaration is often found on the published version of record. Funding is treated similarly.

RevMan 5.4 Tutorial

RevMan is a freely available software tool from Cochrane that allows researchers to build systematic review protocols, full systematic reviews and conduct meta-analyses.

Step 1: Download RevMan v5.4.

```
https://training.cochrane.org/online-learning/core-software-
cochrane-reviews/revman/revman-5-download
```

Select 'for academic use', 'submit', follow prompts over next few pages and then download the software.

Step 2: Developing a research question or aim. The types of questions that can be answered by research are designated 'foreground questions'. Not all questions can be answered by research, and these are background questions. Clinical questions fall into categories of treatment, diagnosis, prognosis and aetiology.

7.6.5 Using the PICO Method

PICO is an acronym for four elements that make up a well-developed research question, namely population, intervention, control and outcomes. Using these four elements enables researchers to formulate researchable questions out of clinical questions. We may be interested in whether maternal supplementation with vitamin A reduces the risk of maternal or child mortality. In this example, the population we are interested in investigating is pregnant women. We could narrow this further if we wished to include only women in a specific region or age group. The intervention is vitamin A supplementation. The control or comparator will be non-supplementation. The outcome that we are interested in is maternal mortality. The outcome is the measure by which we will decide whether the intervention has made any effect on the population. By using this system, we develop 'conceptual buckets', which we can then use when deciding on which search terms to use to find papers that will answer the research question.

Research question/aim:

Does vitamin A supplementation during pregnancy reduce the risk of perinatal morbidity and mortality among pregnant women compared with non-supplementation or controls?

Key: Population Intervention Control Outcome

The outcome that we want to assess is mortality risk.

Step 3: Conducting a systematic search. Inclusion and exclusion criteria:

Inclusion criteria	Exclusion criteria
Studies written in English	Studies not available in English
Full text papers in peer-reviewed journals	Abstracts, conference proceedings and grey literature
Randomised control trials	
Studies on pregnant women	Observational studies/non-intervention study designs
Studies on vitamin A supplementation	Studies on the elderly and men
Maternal mortality as an outcome	Infant mortality or growth as an outcome

Search Terms

$$\left(\left(\left(\left(\left(\text{vitamin A} \right) \text{ OR } \left(\text{retinol} \right) \right) \text{ AND } \left(\text{maternal} \right) \right) \text{ AND } \left(\text{pregnancy} \right) \right) \text{ AND } \left(\text{maternal mortality} \right) \text{ AND } \left(\text{supplementation} \right) \right)$$

This Boolean operator can be pasted directly into the search bar on PubMed. Click 'search'.

https://pubmed.ncbi.nlm.nih.gov

Apply filters to search results for inclusion/exclusion criteria (randomised controlled trials only; full text papers only)

At the top of the page, you are given the option to save the results of the search. Click 'save' and then select 'all results' and 'PubMed' format from the drop-down options. This is important as RevMan can read references in selected formats later when we import the references to the studies, saving a lot of work.

Click create file. PubMed will generate a .txt file (text file for notepad) that will automatically download. Open the file and save it somewhere you will be able to find it later. It is important that the full set of studies is downloaded as you will be able to make decisions on which studies to include in the final meta-analysis and which to exclude.

Next, screen the articles according to your protocol for inclusion in the final meta-analysis. First screen by title, then abstract and finally by full text. Keep notes at each stage as this will be used for your PRISMA flow diagram.

The example I have used here yielded 23 articles from the search (enough for a quick tutorial!). The full references for the articles are provided in Appendix A.

I have screened the articles, and the final studies to include are as follows:

West et al. (1999), Katz et al. (2000), Christian et al. (2000) and Kirkwood et al. (2010).

Step 4: Data extraction. Additionally, for the meta-analysis, we will need some numbers. RevMan will generate a comparison table under Analyses, so we will need the data required for this: the number of study participants who were included in each arm of the study (treatment and control) and the number of study participants who experienced an event during the trial (in this case the number of participants who died).

Another outcome table could be generated by RevMan that includes the means and standard deviations for participants in each treatment arm. For the purposes of this tutorial, we will use the events and total numbers so that RevMan can generate odds ratios.

Outcome 1: Maternal mortality

Study	Treatment (vitamin A supplementation)		Control/no supplementation	
	Events	Total	Events	Total
West et al. (1999)	11	7747	17	7241
West et al. (2011)	Unable to access			
Katz et al. (2000)	9	6070	14	5653
Christian et al. (2000)	23	3715	42	3413
Kirkwood et al. (2010)	138	39601	148	39324
Fawzi et al. (1998)	Unable to access			

Step 5: Importing references to RevMan. We now have the information we need to proceed to RevMan. Open the program and select new review. A window will open that will allow you to name your review. Select the most appropriate format and give the review a title. I have used 'Vitamin A supplementation for preventing maternal mortality: A systematic review and meta-analysis'.

Next, click 'file', then under references, choose 'import'. You will then be shown a window, find the txt file you saved earlier and select 'open'. Click next. The next page of the window will ask you to choose the format of the references file. Since our references are from PubMed, choose the PubMed/MEDLINE format. RevMan will automatically exclude text that is not in the format it is looking for, so you many include your own notes in the txt file without affecting the references. If RevMan tells you that it is excluding many lines of text which are actually references, or that there are no studies found, check that your txt file is in the correct format and try importing again. Click next. The next page asks you to choose the destination for your references. You can select 'included studies' or 'studies awaiting classification' before clicking next, as the next page will allow you to choose the destination manually. You many also choose to set the default destination as 'excluded studies' as there will be fewer included studies than excluded ones.

Since we have already screened our studies for inclusion, we can manually select the reference destination at this point. Once this is done, click finish.

Step 6: Adding data to the references and analysing data. Now we can add our data to the studies. Hover the cursor over the (left hand) panel, where it says 'Data and analyses' and right-click. Select 'add comparison'. A window will open asking you to name your comparison. Let us name this comparison 'Vitamin A supplementation vs control for maternal mortality'. You can add a new comparison table for each outcome you are interested in. Click next. The wizard then asks what you would like to do with the comparison once the wizard is closed. You can add another comparison table immediately (e.g. vitamin A vs control for infant mortality) or add an outcome under the current comparison. Select 'add an outcome under the new comparison' and then click continue.

You can now choose the type of comparison you want to make. Select the dichotomous data type. This will allow you to enter the total number of participants with events and the total number of participants per treatment arm, which is the information we captured from the studies earlier. Selecting the continuous data type will allow you to enter the mean, standard deviation and number of participants in experimental and control groups. Select dichotomous and click next. We now need to name the outcome. I have named it 'maternal mortality'. You can keep the default group names or edit them. Edit the group label 1 (experimental) as 'vitamin A supplementation'. Click next.

The next window will allow you to choose the statistical analysis method that will be applied. For the purposes of this demonstration, we will continue using the default settings – the Mantel–Haenszel statistical model using fixed effects, and our outcome measure will be the odds ratio. However, in this case, a risk ratio would also be suitable. Click next.

The next window will allow you to choose the confidence interval. Choose 95% (the default setting) and click next.

The next window will offer the option to edit what will appear on the graph. For the left-hand graph label, edit to read 'favours vitamin A'. You can choose how the studies will be arranged on the graph, sorting by year of publication, effect size and other variables. Let us choose sort by study ID (the default option) and then click next. The next window will ask you to choose what to do once this wizard has closed. Choose 'edit the new outcome' and click finish.

On the next wizard, you will begin to input the data we captured earlier. Click on the 'add study data' icon and the wizard will appear. The studies we defined as included studies in the previous step will appear in the left-hand options panel. Hold control or shift and click on each of the studies to highlight them for selection and then click finish. The studies you selected will now appear on the comparison table. Enter the values from your table above, and RevMan will automatically generate a forest plot for your data (Figure 7.6).

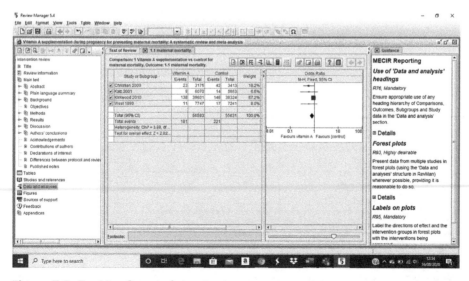

Figure 7.6: RevMan forest plot output.

You can toggle between odds ratio and risk ratio by clicking on the OR icon at the top of the page. Similarly, you can toggle between using fixed and random effect for your model. RevMan will generate an odds ratio for each study and provide details on the weighting of each study. It will also present an estimate of the heterogeneity of the data – in this case a Chi-square with $p = 0.27$ and $I^2 = 23\%$. I^2 less than 25% may be considered to be low heterogeneity, 50% moderate heterogeneity, and 75% a high level of heterogeneity; however, this should be interpreted with caution as it is not an absolute measure of heterogeneity – I^2 reflects variances in effect sizes and does not reflect sampling error. Other researchers suggest simply using $I^2 < 50\%$ as acceptable heterogeneity and $I^2 > 50\%$ as unacceptable.

You will also see that there is a Z-score test for the overall effect, in this case $p = 0.04$.

7.6.5.1 Interpreting the Forest Plot

The blue squares on Figure 7.7 represent the position of the result of each individual study. The horizontal lines represent the 95% CI of the result for each study (short lines mean a smaller confidence interval). The black diamond represents the overall effect of the intervention.

Finally, to answer the research question, it appears that maternal supplementation with vitamin A during pregnancy has a protective effect against maternal mortality ($p = 0.04$); however, this effect is weak (OR = 0.82; 95% CI = 0.67–0.99). This result should be interpreted with caution as the meta-analysis was conducted by one researcher, and there were no controls on bias. In addition, there was only one outcome

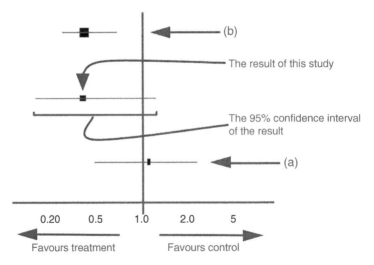

Figure 7.7: Interpreting the forest plot.

assessed – the effect of vitamin A supplementation on maternal mortality. It would be beneficial to determine whether vitamin A supplementation has a positive or negative effect on infant outcomes such as risk of stillbirth or neonatal mortality and morbidity to gain a fuller understanding of the consequences of this intervention.

Appendix A   Studies from Search

Included studies are presented in green, excluded studies in red.

1. West, K.P. Jr., Christian, P., and Labrique, A.B. (2011). Effects of vitamin A or beta carotene supplementation on pregnancy-related mortality and infant mortality in rural Bangladesh: a cluster randomised trial. JAMA 305 (19): 1986–1995. http://dx.doi.org/10.1001/jama.2011.656.
2. Cox, S.E., Arthur, P., and Kirkwood, B.R. (2006). Vitamin A supplementation increases ratios of proinflammatory to anti-inflammatory cytokine responses in pregnancy and lactation. Clin. Exp. Immunol. 144 (3): 392–400. http://dx.doi.org/10.1111/j.1365–2249.2006.03082.x.
3. Labrique, A.B., Christian, P., Klemm, R.D. et al. (2011). A cluster-randomised, placebo-controlled, maternal vitamin A or beta-carotene supplementation trial in Bangladesh: design and methods. Trials 12: 102. http://dx.doi.org/10.1186/1745–6215–12–102.
4. Katz, J., West, K.P. Jr., Khatry, S.K. et al. (2000). Maternal low-dose vitamin A or beta-carotene supplementation has no effect on fetal loss and early infant mortality: a randomized cluster trial in Nepal. Am. J. Clin. Nutr. 71 (6): 1570–1576. http://dx.doi.org/10.1093/ajcn/71.6.1570.
5. Christian, P., West, K.P. Jr., Katz, J. et al. (2004). Cigarette smoking during pregnancy in rural Nepal. Risk factors and effects of beta-carotene and vitamin A supplementation. Eur. J. Clin. Nutr. 58 (2): 204–211. http://dx.doi.org/10.1038/sj.ejcn.1601767.
6. Christian, P., West, K.P., Khatry, S.K. et al. (2003). Effects of maternal micronutrient supplementation on fetal loss and infant mortality: a cluster-randomized trial in Nepal. Am. J. Clin. Nutr. 78 (6): 1194–1202. http://dx.doi.org/10.1093/ajcn/78.6.1194.
7. Christian, P., West, K.P. Jr., Khatry, S.K. et al. (2000). Night blindness during pregnancy and subsequent mortality among women in Nepal: effects of vitamin A and beta-carotene supplementation. Am. J. Epidemiol. 152 (6): 542–547. http://dx.doi.org/10.1093/aje/152.6.542.

8. Kirkwood, B.R., Hurt, L., Amenga-Etego, S. et al. (2010). Effect of vitamin A supplementation in women of reproductive age on maternal survival in Ghana (ObaapaVitA): a cluster-randomised, placebo-controlled trial. Lancet 375 (9726): 1640–1649. https://doi.org/10.1016/S0140-6736(10)60311-X.

9. Prawirohartono, E.P., Nyström, L., Nurdiati, D.S. et al. (2013). The impact of prenatal vitamin A and zinc supplementation on birth size and neonatal survival – a double-blind, randomized controlled trial in a rural area of Indonesia. Int. J. Vitam. Nutr. Res. 83 (1): 14–25. http://dx.doi.org/10.1024/0300-9831/a000141.

10. West, K.P. Jr., Katz, J., Khatry, S.K. et al. (1999). Double blind, cluster randomised trial of low dose supplementation with vitamin A or beta carotene on mortality related to pregnancy in Nepal. The NNIPS-2 study group. BMJ 318 (7183): 570–575. http://dx.doi.org/10.1136/bmj.318.7183.570.

11. Humphrey, J.H., Iliff, P.J., Marinda, E.T. et al. (2006). Effects of a single large dose of vitamin A, given during the postpartum period to HIV-positive women and their infants, on child HIV infection, HIV-free survival, and mortality. J. Infect. Dis. 193 (6): 860–871. http://dx.doi.org/10.1086/500366.

12. Bhutta, Z.A., Rizvi, A., Raza, F. et al. (2009). A comparative evaluation of multiple micronutrient and iron-folic acid supplementation during pregnancy in Pakistan: impact on pregnancy outcomes. Food Nutr. Bull. 30 (4 Suppl): S496–S505. http://dx.doi.org/10.1177/15648265090304S404.

13. van den Broek, N.R., White, S.A., Flowers, C. et al. (2006). Randomised trial of vitamin A supplementation in pregnant women in rural Malawi found to be anaemic on screening by HemoCue. BJOG 113 (5): 569–576. https://doi.org/10.1111/j.1471-0528.2006.00891.x.2006.

14. Muhihi, A., Sudfeld, C.R., Smith, E.R. et al. (2016). Risk factors for small-for-gestational-age and preterm births among 19,269 Tanzanian newborns. BMC Pregnancy Childbirth 16: 110. http://dx.doi.org/10.1186/s12884-016-0900-5.

15. Tielsch, J.M., Rahmathullah, L., Katz, J. et al. (2008). Maternal night blindness during pregnancy is associated with low birthweight, morbidity, and poor growth in South India. J. Nutr. 138 (4): 787–792. http://dx.doi.org/10.1093/jn/138.4.787.

16. Christian, P., Darmstadt, G.L., Wu, L. et al. (2008). The effect of maternal micronutrient supplementation on early neonatal morbidity in rural Nepal: a randomised, controlled, community trial. Arch. Dis. Child. 93 (8): 660–664. http://dx.doi.org/10.1136/adc.2006.114009.

17. Fawzi, W.W., Msamanga, G.I., Hunter, D. et al. (2002). Randomized trial of vitamin supplements in relation to transmission of HIV-1 through breastfeeding and early child mortality. AIDS 16 (14): 1935–1944. http://dx.doi.org/10.1097/00002030-200209270-00011.

18. Sunawang, Utomo, B., Hidayat, A. et al. (2009). Preventing low birthweight through maternal multiple micronutrient supplementation: a cluster-randomized, controlled trial in Indramayu. West Java. Food Nutr. Bull. 30 (4 Suppl): S488–S495. http://dx.doi.org/10.1177/15648265090304S403.

19. Fawzi, W.W., Msamanga, G.I., Spiegelman, D. et al. (1998). Randomised trial of effects of vitamin supplements on pregnancy outcomes and T cell counts in HIV-1-infected women in Tanzania. Lancet 351 (9114): 1477–1482. http://dx.doi.org/10.1016/s0140-6736(98)04197-x.

20. Khavari, N., Jiang, H., Manji, K. et al. (2014). Maternal multivitamin supplementation reduces the risk of diarrhoea among HIV-exposed children through age 5 years. Int. Healt 6 (4): 298–305. http://dx.doi.org/10.1093/inthealth/ihu061 Epub 2014 Aug 30.

21. Fawzi, W.W., Msamanga, G.I., Kupka, R. et al. (2007). Multivitamin supplementation improves hematologic status in HIV-infected women and their children in Tanzania. Am. J. Clin. Nutr. 85 (5): 1335–1343. http://dx.doi.org/10.1093/ajcn/85.5.1335.

22. Katz, J., West, K.P. Jr., Khatry, S.K. et al. (2001). Twinning rates and survival of twins in rural Nepal. Int. J. Epidemiol. 30 (4): 802–807. http://dx.doi.org/10.1093/ije/30.4.802.

23. Fawzi, W.W., Msamanga, G.I., Wei, R. et al. (2003). Effect of providing vitamin supplements to human immunodeficiency virus-infected, lactating mothers on the child's morbidity and CD4+ cell counts. Clin. Infect. Dis. 36 (8): 1053–1062. http://dx.doi.org/10.1086/374223 Epub 2003 Apr 2.

References

Albarqouni, L., Hoffmann, T., Strauss, S. et al. (2018). Core competencies in evidence-based practice for health professionals consensus statement based on a systematic review and Delphi survey. *JAMA Netw. Open* 1 (2): e180281.

Bajaj, J.K., Salwan, P., and Salwan, S. (2016). Various possible toxicants involved in thyroid dysfunction: a review. *J. Clin. Diagn. Res.* 10 (1): FE01–FE03.

Baliki, G., Bruck, T., Schreinemachers, P., and Uddin, M.N. (2019). Long-term behavioural impact of an integrated home garden intervention: evidence from Bangladesh. *Food Secur.* 11: 1217–1230.

Bernal, J. (2005). Thyroid hormones and brain development. *Vitam. Horm.* 71: 95–122.

Correa-Agudelo, E., Kim, H.Y., Musuka, G.N. et al. (2021). The epidemiological landscape of anemia in women of reproductive age in sub-Saharan Africa. *Sci. Rep.* 11: 11955.

De Benoist, B., Andersson, M., Egli, I. et al. (2004). *Iodine Status Worldwide: WHO Global Database on Iodine Deficiency*. Geneva: World Health Organisation.

De Escobar, G.M., Obregion, M.J., and del Rey, F.E. (2004). Role of thyroid hormone during early brain development. *Eur. J. Endocrinol.* 151: 25–37.

Eastman, C.J. and Zimmermann, M.B. (2000). The iodine deficiency disorders. In: *Endotext* (ed. K.R. Feingold, B. Anawalt, A. Boyce, et al.). South Dartmouth, MA, USA: http://MDText.com, Inc. https://www.ncbi.nlm.nih.gov/books/NBK285556.

Faber, M., Venter, S.J., and Spinnler Benade, A.J. (2002). Increased vitamin A intake in children aged 2–5 years through targeted home-gardens in a rural south African community. *Public Health Nutr.* 5 (1): 11–16.

Fuge, R. and Johnson, C.C. (2015). Iodine and human health, the role of environmental geochemistry and diet, a review. *Appl. Geochem.* 63: 282–302.

Goddard, A.F., James, M.W., McIntyre, A.S. et al. (2011). Guidelines for the management of iron deficiency anaemia. *Gut* 60: 1309–1316.

Lazarus, J.H. (2015). The importance of iodine in public health. *Environ. Geochem. Health* 37: 605–618.

Lei, J., Nowbar, S., Mariash, C.N., and Ingbar, D.H. (2003). Thyroid hormone stimulates Na-K- ATPase activity and its plasma membrane insertion in rat alveolar epithelial cells. *Am. J. Physiol. Lung Cell. Mol. Physiol.* 285 (3): 762–772.

Lodish, H., Berk, A., Zipursky, S.L. et al. (2000). *Molecular Cell Biology* (Section 15.5, Active Transport by ATP-Powered Pumps), 4e. New York: W. H. Freeman https://www.ncbi.nlm.nih.gov/books/NBK21481.

Minihane, A.M. and Rimbach, G. (2002). Iron absorption and the iron binding and anti-oxidant properties of phytic acid. *Int. J. Food Sci. Technol.* 37: 741–748.

Prieto-Patron, A., Van der Horst, K., Hutton, Z.V., and Detzel, P. (2018). Association between anaemia in children 6 to 23 months old and child, mother, household and feeding indicators. *Nutrients* 10 (9): 1269.

Roy, A., Fuentes-Afflick, E., Fernald, L.C.H., and Young, S.L. (2018). Pica is prevalent and strongly associated with iron deficiency among Hispanic pregnant women living in the United States. *Appetite* 120: 163–170.

West, C.E. and Castenmiller, J.J. (1998). Quantification of the "SLAMENGHI" factors for carotenoid bioavailability and bioconversion. *Int. J. Vitam. Nutr. Res.* 68 (6): 371–377.

World Health Organisation (2008). *Worldwide Prevalence of Anaemia 1993–2005*. Geneva: WHO.

Young, G.P., Mortimer, E.K., Gopalsamy, G.L. et al. (2014). Zinc deficiency in children with environmental enteropathy-development of new strategies: report from an expert workshop. *Am. J. Clin. Nutr.* 100 (4): 1198–1207.

Zimmerman, M.B. and Boelaert, K. (2015). Iodine deficiency and thyroid disorders. *Lancet Diabetes Endocrinol.* 3 (4): 286–295.

Zimpita, T., Biggs, C., and Faber, M. (2015). Gardening practices in a rural village in South Africa 10 years after completion of a home garden project. *Food Nutr. Bull.* 36 (1): 33–42.

WHO and FAO (2006). *Guidelines on food fortification with micronutrients.* Geneva: World Health Organisation.

Castejon, H.V., Ortega, P., Amaya, D. et al. (2013). Co-existence of anaemia, vitamin A deficiency and growth retardation among children 24-84 months old in Maracaibo, Venezuela. *Nutritional Neuroscience* 7 (2): 113–119.

Sazawal, S., Black, R.E., Ramsan, M. et al. (2006). Effects of routine prophylactic supplementation with iron and folic acid on admission to hospital and mortality in preschool children in a high malaria transmission setting: community-based, randomised, placebo-controlled trial. *Lancet* 367 (9505): 133–143.

Caulfield, L.E. and Black, R.E. (2004). Zinc deficiency. Comparative quantification of health risks: global and regional burden of disease attributable to selected major risk factors. *World Health Org* 1: 257–280.

Berhe, K., Gebrearegay, F., and Gebremariam, H. (2019). Prevalence and associated factors of zinc deficiency among pregnant women and children in Ethiopia: A systematic review and meta-analysis. *BMC Public Health* 19: 1663.

Smith, M.R., DeFries, R., Chhatre, A. et al. (2019). Inadequate zinc intake in India: Past, present and future. *Food Nutr Bull* 40 (1): 26–40.

Barth-Jaeggi, T., Moretti, D., Kvalsvig, J. et al. (2016). In-home fortification with 2.5 mg iron as NaFeEDTA does not reduce anaemia but increases weight gain: A randomised controlled trial in Kenyan infants. *Maternal and Child Nutrition* 11 (S4): 151–162.

Nuss, E.T. and Tanumihardjo, S.A. (2016). Maize: A paramount staple crop in the context of global nutrition. *Comprehensive Reviews in Food Science and Food Safety* 9 (4): 417–436.

Gebremedhin, S. (2017). Vitamin A supplementation and childhood morbidity from diarrhea, fever, respiratory problems and anemia in sub-Saharan Africa. *Nutrition and Dietary Supplements* 9: 47–54.

De Groote, H., Kimenju, S.C., and Morawetz, U.B. (2010). Estimating consumer willingness to pay for food quality with experimental auctions: The case of yellow versus fortified maize meal in Kenya. *Agricultural Economics* 42 (1): 1–16.

Grellety, E. and Golden, M.H. (2016). The effect of random error on diagnostic accuracy illustrated with the anthropometric diagnosis of malnutrition. *PLoS ONE* 11 (12): e0168585.

Kennedy, G., Nantel, G., and Shetty, P. (2003). The "scourge" of hidden hunger: Global dimensions of micronutrient deficiencies. *Food Nutrition and Agriculture* 32: 8–16.

Mayer, J.E., Pfeiffer, W.H., and Beyer, P. (2008). Bio-fortified crops to alleviate micronutrient malnutrition. *Journal of Current Opinion in Plant Biology* 11 (2): 166–170.

FAO (2003). *Food, Nutrition and Agriculture.* Geneva, FAO: ISSN 1014-806X.

Codija, G. (2001). Food sources of vitamin A and provitamin A specific to Africa: an FAO perspective. *Food and Nutrition Bulletin* 22 (6): https://doi.org/10.1177/156482650102200403.

IVACG (2003). *Improving the vitamin A status of populations*. Washington, USA: Report of the XXI IVACG.

Mason, J., Greiner, T., Shrimpton, R. et al. (2015). Vitamin A policies need rethinking. *International Journal of Epidemiology* 44 (1): 283–292.

WHO (2009). Global prevalence of vitamin A deficiency in populations at risk 1995-2005. In: *WHO Global Database on Vitamin A Deficiency*. Geneva: World Health Organisation.

World Health Organisation, Centers for Disease Control and Prevention (2008). Worldwide prevalence of anaemia 1993-2005. In: *WHO Global Database on Anaemia* (ed. B. Benoist, E. McLean, I. Egil and M. Cogswell). Geneva: World Health Organisation.

8 The Nutritional Double Burden of Disease

8.1 Introduction

The nutritional double burden of disease refers to the phenomenon of undernutrition, wasting, stunting, micronutrient deficiency coinciding with overweight, obesity, and diet-related non-communicable diseases within individuals, households and populations throughout the life cycle (WHO 2017).

The nutritional double burden of disease is becoming a major health problem in low- and middle-income countries, especially among children (Tzioumis and Adair 2014). Sub-Saharan African countries with a high prevalence of childhood undernutrition have a correspondingly high prevalence of adult undernutrition, not indicative of the nutritional double burden (Wojcicki 2014). However, while stunting, underweight and wasting caused by undernutrition remain prevalent in developing countries (De Onis et al. 2011), the prevalence of overweight and obesity is increasing (Figure 8.1). Studies conducted in South Africa suggest the existence of a nutritional double burden of disease, in which both under- and overnutrition are found in the same communities, households and even in individuals (Tzioumis and Adair 2014). Evidence of the double burden of disease is being found in both urban and rural areas of the country (Kimani-Murage 2013).

8.2 Causes of the Nutritional Double Burden

Infection, diet quality and physical activity levels coupled with anaemia and other underlying factors that are associated with stunting and overweight may occur simultaneously in the same individual (Tzioumis and Adair 2014). A nutritional double burden effect, which has been linked to the nutrition transition, is the concurrent increasing prevalence

Nutrition and Global Health, First Edition. Shawn W. McLaren.
© 2023 John Wiley & Sons Ltd. Published 2023 by John Wiley & Sons Ltd.

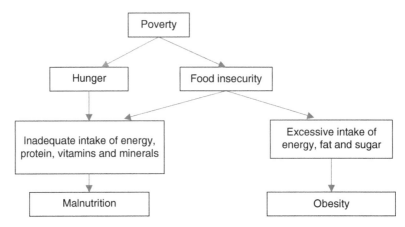

Figure 8.1: The obesity paradox (Whitney and Rolfes 2019).

of overweight women and underweight children (Kruger et al. 2012). Dieffenbach and Stein (2012) have suggested that this problem is partly caused by easy accessibility to energy-dense foods, which are linked with adult overweight and poor accessibility to the nutrient-dense foods that are required for optimal child growth in the same households. In a study conducted in the South–West border area of Texas, an area with high rates of poverty, obesity and household food insecurity, Sharkey et al. (2012) found that very low food security was associated with increased energy, fat and added sugar consumption among children aged between 6 and 11 years. Micronutrient intake of calcium, sodium, potassium, and vitamin D as well as dietary fibre among these children was found to be much lower than the recommended amounts for age (Sharkey et al. 2012).

The nutritional double burden is thought to be driven by three main factors – the nutrition transition, the epidemiological transition and the population transition.

The nutrition transition describes a shift in dietary patterns, consumption and energy expenditure and is associated with economic development over time. Increasing globalisation improves access to new markets. Urbanisation in developing countries increases incomes and access to processed foods. The consequence of the nutrition transition is a shift from a predominance of undernutrition in populations to higher rates of overweight, obesity and non-communicable diseases.

Changes in eating behaviours and physical activity levels con-tribute to the increasing prevalence of obesity in dual-burden coun-tries (Ramachandran 2011). Ramachandran (2011) reported that there was an increase in per capita total energy, protein and fat intake but a reduction in micronutrient intake in India between 1975 and 1996. This phenomenon coincided with an 18% fall in rural areas and 22% in urban areas in per capita expenditure on food. It was suggested that this was caused by a fall in expenditure on cereals as well as the low cost of cereals, especially subsidised cereals, in low-income groups (Ramachandran 2011). Similarly, South African dietary patterns have changed over the past few decades. Goedecke et al. (2005) reported that carbohydrate consumption among South African adults living in urban areas decreased by 10.9% between 1940 and 1990, while fat intake increased by 59.7%. In comparison, fat intake among South African adults in rural areas increased by only 8%, while carbohydrate intake decreased by 10% between 1970 and 1990 (Goedecke et al. 2005).

The epidemiological transition is the change in overall population disease burden associated with the increase in economic prosperity. It is a shift from a predominance of infection and diseases related to undernutrition to rising rates of non-communicable diseases (NCDs).

The population transition is the shift in population structure and lengthening lifespans. This sees a transformation from populations with high birth rates and death rates (related to the above transitions), with relatively high proportions of younger people, to populations with increasing proportions of older people (with age also being a risk factor for many NCDs).

Popkin and Gorden-Larson (2004) have illustrated the phenomenon of the nutrition transition as shown in Figure 8.2. The figure follows a population from a period of receding famine to one which has a high rate of nutrition related chronic diseases of lifestyle. Many low- and middle-income countries are currently making the change from stage 3 in the figure to stage 4.

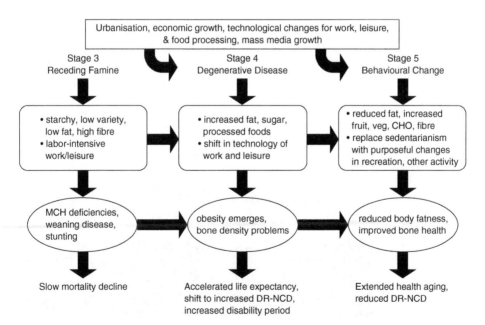

Figure 8.2: Stages of the nutrition transition (Popkin and Gordon-Larson 2004).

8.3 Drivers of the Nutritional Double Burden

Behavioural, social and demographic, biological and environmental factors all contribute to driving the nutritional double burden (Figure 8.3). Among the biological factors is epigenetics. It is thought that intrauterine growth restriction resulting from poor maternal nutrition during or before gestation leads to changes in the way that the infant's body regulates energy. Alterations in the expression of genes are thought to influence the risk of low birthweight, overweight, obesity and non-communicable disease. These changes can be passed on between generations, even once undernutrition is no longer present (Walker et al. 2015).

8.3.1 Early Life Nutrition

Early life nutrition has significant and lifelong impacts on health. The quality and quantity of nutrients and food available during foetal development and infancy affect health outcomes throughout the life cycle.

The obesity epidemic may find its roots in both genetic and environmental causes (Burgio et al. 2015). Restricted dietary intake during pregnancy can alter gene expression in the foetus, which has implications

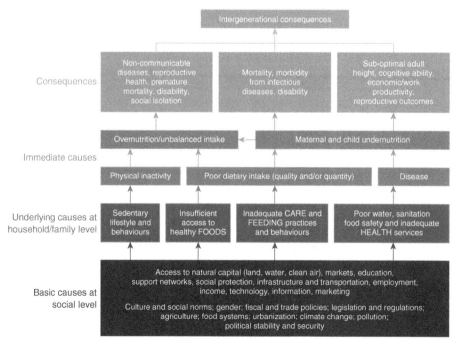

Figure 8.3: WHO conceptual framework on the double burden of disease.

for weight gain and non-communicable disease risk throughout the life cycle. In addition, these epigenetic effects may be passed on to following generations, with evidence emerging that methylation of genes involved in metabolic functions may be found in later generations (Burgio et al. 2015). These effects may be exacerbated by the post-partum environment, particularly when considering the effects of exposure to 'obesogens', chemicals that disrupt hormonal mechanisms for maintaining energy balance (Burgio et al. 2015).

8.4 Regulation of Energy Storage and Expenditure – Including Fat Stores

The risk of serious problems including maternal anaemia and preterm birth and low birthweight increases among women of childbearing age with poor nutritional intake. Low birthweight can increase the risk of chronic diseases of lifestyle and increased abdominal obesity in later stages of the life cycle. Low-birthweight children are at a higher risk of stunting in childhood (McLaren et al. 2018). Stunting is associated with a reduction in fat oxidation and resting energy expenditure (Hoffman et al. 2000a), which is a possible explanation for the increased risk of overweight and obesity among these children later in life. Conversely, the same researchers found that there was no association between stunting and total energy expenditure when differences in body sizes and composition between stunted and non-stunted children were included in the model (Hoffman et al. 2000b), with one exception. Boys had a higher total energy expenditure than girls, which could explain the increased risk of obesity among stunted adolescent girls in urban areas of developing countries (Hoffman et al. 2000b).

Women of childbearing age who are overweight or gain excessive weight during pregnancy are at a higher risk of developing gestational diabetes. Gestational diabetes is associated with higher birthweight infants. These high-birthweight infants are at a greater risk of overweight and obesity later in life.

8.4.1 Accelerated Weight Gain Early in Life Associated with Higher Body Mass Index and Obesity Later in Life

Successful catch-up growth achieved within the first two years of life in stunted children was related to a higher than standard BMI and body fat percentage at the age of five years (Pomeroy et al. 2014; Ong et al. 2000). Evidence suggests that catch-up-growth-related overweight persists into adolescence and adulthood (Kruger et al. 2014). Poor early childhood growth has been suggested as a reason for the increasing burden of obesity (Ong et al. 2000).

8.4.2 Food Access and Portion Sizes

Industrialisation of the food industry during the twentieth century has led to profound changes in the quality and quantity of available foods. This in turn has resulted in major changes in the nutritional status of populations.

The portion sizes of many packaged, restaurant and take-away snacks and meals have increased, while their relative costs have decreased. Concurrently, the cost of fresh produce has increased – particularly among poor consumers in low- and middle-income countries and countries importing food.

Low- and middle-income countries have experienced rapid changes in their agricultural systems, and the introduction of modern retail and food service sectors and the modern food system has penetrated all sectors of the population (Popkin 2015). This has resulted in dietary shifts towards more refined carbohydrates, an increase in added sweeteners and edible oils, more animal source foods and a reduction in the consumption of legumes, vegetables and fruit (Popkin 2015). According to Bosa (2015), West Africa is in the early stages of the nutrition transition. Foods are predominantly traditional, and the major food groups are consumed in their recommended amounts; however, the diet is still generally low in fruit and vegetables and high in energy, fats, sugars and protein. Southern Africa is also experiencing the nutrition transition, where 31–75% of people do not exercise regularly and 72% are not meeting the recommendations for vegetable and fruit intake (Nnyepi et al. 2015).

8.4.3 Socio-economic Disadvantage, Inequality and Poverty

Malnutrition is intimately related to poverty and disease. Low socio-economic status reduces an individual's ability to afford nutrient-rich foods, predisposing them to undernutrition as well as overweight and obesity. There is a correlation between food insecurity, poverty and obesity. The prevalence of overweight and obesity correlates with socio-economic status in middle- and high-income countries. However, obesity is now affecting countries from all wealth categories. Although we find the highest age-standardised prevalence of overweight in the upper-middle income countries, there is also a prevalence of 10–30% of overweight and obesity in low- and middle-income countries.

8.4.4 Urbanisation, Urban Design and the Built Environment

It is estimated that 55% of the world population lives in urban environments, with as many as 50% of people in low- and middle-income countries living in urban settings (World Bank 2020). Urbanisation and economic growth can result in improvements in the nutritional status of populations, but they can also be a significant factor in worsening nutritional status. The latter is particularly relevant for countries and regions in the fourth stage of the nutrition transition.

In urban environments where infrastructure, water and sanitation are inadequate, people are at a higher risk of contracting water-borne diseases, which result in malnutrition. Infectious diseases that result from poor hygiene and sanitation and poor water quality are among significant contributors to anaemia. Micronutrient deficiency is one of the hallmark features of the double burden of malnutrition.

The other mark of the nutritional double burden of disease, features of overnutrition such as overweight and obesity, are also encouraged by the design of urban environments. Urban design and the built environment can discourage physical activity and active travel as people make more use of public transport or motor vehicles for travel and participate in more sedentary jobs and recreational activities.

Food access is also fundamentally affected by urban living. Urbanisation leads to a reduced reliance on smallholder and home-grown foods and a greater reliance on obtaining foods from other suppliers and supply chains, which has an impact on food security. In combination with this, urbanisation comes with an improved access to unhealthy foods, industrial food systems and food advertising. These aspects of urbanisation influence increase the risk of overweight and obesity, and disproportionately affect the poor.

The contrast between urban and rural dietary composition puts urbanisation at the forefront of the causes of the nutrition transition taking place in the developing world. However, more recent studies have shown that the effects of the nutrition transition are becoming more prevalent in rural areas as well. Kimani-Murage (2013) showed that stunting and overweight coexist in rural South African communities, particularly affecting girls. Pedro et al. (2014) discovered high rates of glucose intolerance and pre-hypertension among rural South African adolescents. Igumbor et al. (2012) suggested that rapid urbanisation and monopolies on food production and distribution are significant factors in the nutrition transition in South Africa. Processed and prepared foods are generally high in calories, fat and salt. These foods are rapidly becoming more affordable, accessible and acceptable to all populations in South Africa, including rural and informal settlements (Igumbor et al. 2012). Unexpectedly, high proportions of South Africans living in rural areas purchase their food from supermarkets, perhaps explaining the presence of the nutritional double burden in rural as well as urban communities (D'Haese and Huylenbroek 2005). Changes in sales volumes of processed and convenience foods reveal that sales of these foods increased dramatically in South Africa between 2005 and 2010 (Igumbor et al. 2012).

8.4.4.1 Overweight and Obesity

The prevalence of obesity has doubled in over 70 countries since 1980 (The GBD 2015 Obesity Collaborators 2015). Both adult and child populations have been affected. The prevalence of obesity is lower among children than adults; however, the rate of increase in obesity prevalence is far higher among children (The GBD 2015 Obesity Collaborators 2015).

The prevalence of overweight and obesity among children is increasing. The global prevalence of childhood overweight and obesity increased from 4.2 to 6.7% between 1990 and 2010 (De Onis et al. 2011). De Onis et al. (2011) estimate the global prevalence to reach 60 million by 2020. Of the estimated 43 million overweight and obese children worldwide, 35 million were from developing countries (De Onis et al. 2011). In one study, 8.5% of African children were estimated to be overweight or obese (De Onis et al. 2011). Overweight was prevalent among 7.4% and obesity among 2.5% of children between 7 and 14 years old ($n = 445$) in Ethiopia (Wolde et al. 2015).

The consequences of this rapid rise in obesity rates include higher rates of morbidity and mortality. Obesity contributed to 120 million disability-adjusted life years, contributing 5% of all disability-adjusted life years from any cause among adults (The GBD 2015 Obesity Collaborators 2015).

8.4.4.1.1 Defining Overweight and Obesity Overweight and obesity are 'conditions of abnormal or excessive fat accumulation in adipose tissue, to the extent that health may be impaired' (Garrow 1988). The underlying disease is the undesirable positive energy balance and weight gain.

Obesity is measured using body mass index (BMI). Development and use of this index are described in further detail in Chapter 2. The index is based on weight and height and can be measured and calculated with simple equipment and does not necessarily require specialist knowledge to calculate and interpret. The tool is considered accurate and reliable. In addition, BMI values are comparable for males and females and across ages in adults, making it a useful tool for clinical as well as epidemiological

Table 8.1: WHO (2004) BMI classifications.

BMI	Classification	Risk of co-morbidities
25–29.9 kg/m²	Overweight	Increased
30–34.9 kg/m²	Obese class I	Moderate
35–39.9 kg/m²	Obese class II	Severe
>40 kg/m²	Obese class III	Very severe

work. BMI is closely associated with the risk of morbidity and mortality, particularly with type 2 diabetes in higher BMI categories and respiratory diseases in lower categories. However, an important limitation is that it does not differentiate fat mass (FM) from fat-free mass (FFM). This is significant as it may result in misclassification of individuals based on body FM and percentage. There is heterogeneity in the amount of excess fat stored by obese individuals, and importantly, differences in the regional distribution of body fat (Garrow 1988). The distribution of adipose tissue around the body has a strong influence on the risks associated with obesity (Garrow 1988). Other indicators of body composition are more accurate, but are also more costly, complicated and invasive. Waist circumference is a useful indicator of excess abdominal adiposity (Table 8.1).

8.4.4.2 Energy Balance

The energy balance can be presented as an equation that always balances:

$$[\text{Nutrient intake}] - [\text{nutrient utilisation}] = [\text{change in body nutrient stores}]$$

If energy intake is greater than energy utilisation, then there will be a corresponding increase in body energy stores. If energy intake is less than utilisation, the result will be a diminishing of body energy stores. Dietary carbohydrate, fat and protein contribute to energy intake. The body stores a small amount of carbohydrate in the form of glycogen and blood glucose, protein is stored in lean tissues and forms the nitrogen pool, and fats are stored in adipose tissue. Energy expenditure is made up of basal metabolism, thermogenesis and physical activity. The largest proportion of energy expenditure comes from basal metabolism. This is the energy required for maintaining essential body functions. Protein turnover and maintaining cellular concentrations of salts through the action of Na K ATPase pumps (see Chapter 6) account for the largest contribution to the basal metabolic rate. Fat-free mass is metabolically

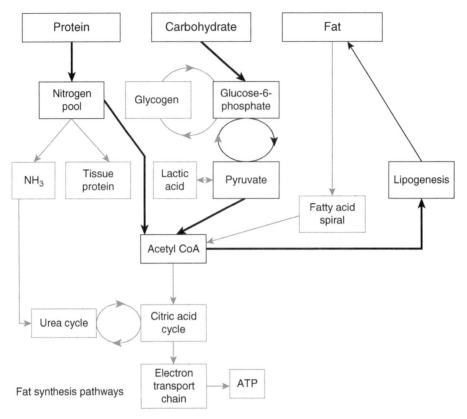

Figure 8.4: Macronutrient conversion to fat.

active tissue, whereas FM is relatively metabolically inert. (Donelly and Smith 2005).

Macronutrients can all be converted to fatty acids (Figure 8.4). Therefore, the excessive intake of any or all macronutrients can contribute to excess adiposity. Carbohydrate and protein have lower energy density (4 kcal/g) than fat (9 kcal/g). Carbohydrates have a greater utilisation rate than proteins or fats. Set point theory refers to the active, biological control of body weight at a set point (Muller et al. 2010).

8.4.4.3 Regulation of Energy Intake

Hunger, appetite and satiety are regulated physiologically by the hypothalamus, stomach, adipose tissue and liver (Figure 8.5). Satiety is influenced by the size of a meal and the individual's appetite. Nutritional quality of the meal can also influence satiety.

Prior to a meal, the stomach produces the hormone ghrelin which stimulates appetite. During a meal, insulin is released which suppresses lipolysis and stimulates lipogenesis, increasing the number of fatty acids taken up by the cells. Once adipose tissue begins to fill with free fatty

CONTROL OF FOOD INTAKE

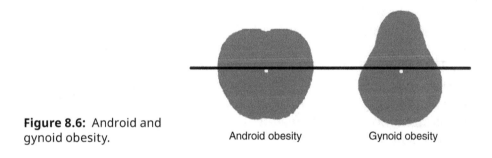

Figure 8.5: Control of food intake.

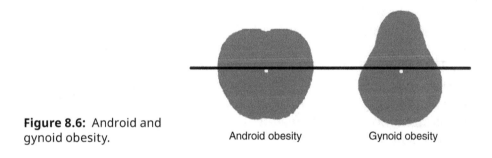

Figure 8.6: Android and gynoid obesity.

acids, leptin is released from the adipocytes, which suppresses appetite by signalling to the hypothalamus that the individual can stop eating.

It has been observed that hypothalamic leptin sensitivity is diminished in obese individuals, leading to leptin resistance and diminished anorexic effect of this hormone (Gruzdeva et al. 2019). In addition, high fructose corn syrup, a common ingredient in many processed foods, does not result in a significant insulin or leptin secretion, therefore not contributing to satiety but contributing to energy intake (Basciano et al. 2005).

In subjects with CAD, including those with normal and high BMI, central obesity but not BMI is associated with mortality (Figure 8.6). Mortality risks associated with different types of obesity are presented in Table 8.2.

8.4.5 Obesity and Poor Iron Status

Concurrent under- and overnutrition is a feature of the double burden of malnutrition. This may affect communities, households and individuals. An individual may display signs of overnutrition, such as overweight

Table 8.2: Mortality risk and obesity type.

Type of obesity	Mortality risk (HR)
Central obesity	1.70 (95% CI 1.58–1.83)
High BMI	0.64 (95% CI 0.59–0.69)
Normal BMI but central obesity	1.70 (95% CI: 1.52–1.89)

and obesity, and simultaneously suffer from micronutrient deficiencies. This may be due to poor quality diets, which are high in energy and fat, but micronutrient poor, or perhaps because of more sedentary lifestyles as work involves less physical activity. There may also be physiological processes that link obesity and poor micronutrient status. In terms of iron status, there has been speculation that inflammatory processes resulting from overweight and obesity interrupt normal iron homeostasis. People with overweight, obesity or the metabolic syndrome display a chronic, low-intensity inflammatory response (Rogero and Calder 2018). This obesity-related inflammation is mediated by the toll-like receptor 4 (TLR4) pathway. It appears that saturated fatty acids activate the TLR4 pathway, resulting in inflammation. Polyunsaturated fats exert the opposite effect (Rogero and Calder 2018). Hepcidin production is affected by the presence of pro-inflammatory cytokines. Hepcidin binds with ferroportin at the site of iron absorption, resulting in its destruction. Excess hepcidin production may result in low ferritin saturation and transferrin binding saturation, in spite of a diet that is adequate in iron.

8.4.6 Causes of Obesity

Unmodifiable causes of obesity involve an interaction between the environment and an individual's predisposition to overweight and obesity. The conceptual framework on the causes of obesity developed by Ang et al. (2013) describes this interaction between genetics, the intrauterine environment and ethnicity with an obesogenic environment as causative factors for childhood obesity (Figure 8.7). Factors including maternal obesity, weight gain during gestation, gestational diabetes, the intrauterine environment and epigenetics are all characteristics related to maternal or women of childbearing age health that play a role in childhood overweight and obesity.

Modifiable risk factors for increases in children's BMI, body weight and adiposity stem from parental determinants and socio-economic factors. Among children under five years living in rural South African areas, overweight was associated with an irregular source of household income (Lesiapeto et al. 2010).

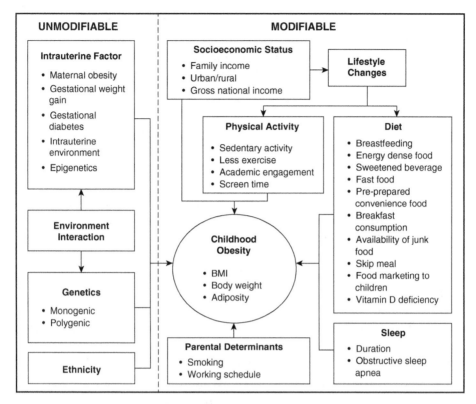

Figure 8.7: Conceptual framework of the causes of obesity (Ang et al. 2013).

8.4.7 Prevention/Treatment of Obesity in Children

Interventions aimed at reducing overweight and obesity should be directed towards pre-adolescent and adolescent girls, as this population group displays high levels of overweight and obesity in rural South Africa (Craig et al. 2015).

However, according to a systematic review on the effectiveness of interventions into childhood overweight, none of the interventions reviewed had any effect on preventing childhood overweight and obesity (Monasta et al. 2011).

8.4.8 Strategies to Address the Double Burden of Malnutrition

The problem of the nutritional double burden of malnutrition has been discussed in the literature for decades. However, the two main features of the double burden of malnutrition – under- and overnutrition – largely continue to be investigated separately. Policies and programmes aim to address either stunting and underweight or overweight but rarely aim to address both simultaneously. Therefore, there is a lack of evidence on effective 'double duty actions' – policies and interventions that are capable of simultaneously addressing under- and overnutrition (Nugent et al. 2020).

Intervention strategies for the double burden of malnutrition focus on either addressing underweight or overweight, with few examples of effective 'double duty actions' available in the literature (Menon and Penalvo 2020). Interventions addressing undernutrition typically focus on poverty reduction, while interventions addressing overweight and obesity tend to focus on nutrition education and physical activity (Menon and Penalvo 2020). One area of overlap is school feeding schemes. Sekiyama et al. (2017) investigated a school lunch intervention that focused on sustainable foods. The intervention resulted in improvements in iron status and anthropometry among children who were undernourished at the start of the intervention, but no changes were observed among overweight children (Sekiyama et al. 2017). A study in Burkino Faso aimed to address the double burden of malnutrition through an innovative school feeding scheme (Edde et al. 2019). It was found that thinness was positively impacted by the intervention, but there was no effect on overweight and obesity (Edde et al. 2019). Nutrition-sensitive interventions including cash transfers have been proposed to address the underlying causes of the double burden of malnutrition. Conkin et al. (2018) modelled the effects of increasing minimum wages in 24 low- and middle-income countries on the nutritional status of women. The model showed a positive correlation between earnings and weight gain among malnourished women, but increasing incomes did not have a protective effect against overweight and obesity (Conkin et al. 2018). Given that there is a lack of evidence for 'double-duty' interventions, a plausible approach is to identify under- or overnutrition in communities for referral to an appropriate intervention for either under- or overnutrition.

References

Ang, Y.N., Wee, B.S., Poh, B.K., and Ismail, M.N. (2013). Multifactorial influences of childhood obesity. *Curr. Obes. Rep.* 2: 10–22.

Basciano, H., Federico, L., and Adeli, K. (2005). Fructose, insulin resistance and metabolic dyslipidaemia. *Nutr. Metab. (Lond.)* 2: 5.

Bosa, K. (2015). An overview of the nutrition transition in West Africa: implications for non-communicable diseases. *Proc. Nutr. Soc.* 74 (4): 466–477.

Burgio, E., Lopomo, A., and Migliore, L. (2015). Obesity and diabetes: from genetics to epigenetics. *Mol. Biol. Rep.* https://doi.org/10.1007/s11033-014-3751-z.

Conkin, A.I., Ponce, N.A., Crespi, C.M. et al. (2018). Economic policy and the double burden of malnutrition: cross-national longitudinal analysis of minimum wage and women's underweight and obesity. *Public Health Nutr.* 21 (5): 940–947.

Craig, E., Reilly, J.J., and Bland, R. (2015). Risk factors for overweight and overfatness in rural South African children and adolescents. *J. Public Health* 38 (1): 24–33.

De Onis, M., Blossner, M., and Borghi, E. (2011). Prevalence and trends of stunting among pre-school children 1990–2020. *Public Health Nutr.* 15 (1): 142–148.

D'Haese, M. and Huylenbroek, G.V. (2005). The rise of supermarkets and changing expenditure patterns of rural households case study in the Transkei area, South Africa. *Food Policy* 30: 97–113.

Dieffenbach, S. and Stien, A.D. (2012). Stunted child/overweight mother pairs represent a statistical artefact, not a distinct entity. *J. Nutr.* 142 (4): 771–773.

Donelly, J.E. and Smith, B.K. (2005). Is exercise effective for weight loss with ad libitum diet? Energy balance, compensation, and gender differences. *Exerc. Sport Sci. Rev.* 33 (4): 169–174.

Edde, E.C., Delisle, H., Dabone, C., and Batal, M. (2019). Impact of the Nutrition-Friendly School Initiative: Analysis of anthropometric and biochemical data among school-aged children in Ouagadougou. *Glob. Health Promot.* EPub.

Garrow, J.S. (1988). *Obesity and Related Diseases*, 1–16. London: Churchill Livingstone.

Goedecke JH, Jennings CL, Lambert EU (2005). Obesity in South Africa. Chronic Diseases of Lifestyle since 1995: 65-79.

Gruzdeva, O., Borodkina, D., Uchasova, E. et al. (2019). Leptin resistance: underlying mechanisms and diagnosis. *Diabetes Metab. Syndr. Obes.* 12: 191–198.

Hoffman, D.J., Sawaya, A.L., Verreschi, I. et al. (2000a). Why are nutritionally stunted children at increased risk of obesity? Studies of metabolic rate and fat oxidation in shantytown children from Sao Paulo, Brazil. *Am. J. Clin. Nutr.* 72 (3): 702–707.

Hoffman, D.J., Sawaya, A.L., Coward, W.A. et al. (2000b). Energy expenditure of stunted and nonstunted boys and girls living in the shantytowns of Sao Paulo, Brazil. *Am. J. Clin. Nutr.* 72 (4): 1025–1031.

Igumbor, E.U., Sanders, D., Puoane, T.R. et al. (2012). 'Big Food,' the consumer food environment, health, and the policy response in South Africa. *PLoS Med.* 9 (7): e1001253.

Kimani-Murage, E.W. (2013). Exploring the paradox: double burden of malnutrition in rural South Africa. *Glob. Health Action* 6: 193–205.

Kruger, H.S., Steyn, N.P., Swart, E.C. et al. (2012). Overweight among children decreased, but obesity prevalence remained high among women in South Africa, 1999–2005. *Public Health Nutr.* 15 (4): 594–599.

Kruger, G., Pienaar, A.E., Coetzee, D., and Kruger, S.H. (2014). Prevalence of stunting, wasting and underweight in Grade 1-learners: The NE-CHILD study. *Health SA Gesondheid* 19 (1): 1–7.

Lesiapeto, M.S., Smuts, C.M., Hanekom, S.M. et al. (2010). Risk factors of poor anthropometric status in children under five years of age living in rural districts of the Eastern Cape and KwaZulu-Natal provinces, South Africa. *S. Afr. J. Clin. Nutr.* 23 (4): 202–207.

McLaren, S., Steenkamp, L., Feeley, A. et al. (2018). Food insecurity, social welfare and low birth weight: implications for childhood malnutrition in an urban eastern Cape Province township. *S. Afr. J. Child Health* 12 (3): 95–99. ISSN 1999-7671.

Menon, S. and Penalvo, J.L. (2020). Actions targeting the double burden of malnutrition: A scoping review. *Nutrients* 12 (1): 81.

Monasta, L., Batty, G.D., Macaluso, A. et al. (2011). Interventions for the prevention of overweight and obesity in preschool children: a systematic review of randomized controlled trials. *Obes. Rev.* 12 (5): e107–e118.

Muller, M.J., Bosy-Westphal, A., and Heymsfield, S.B. (2010). Is there evidence for a set point that regulates human body weight? *F1000 Med. Rep.* 2 (59): https://doi.org/10.3410%2FM2-59.

Nugent, R., Levin, C., Hale, J., and Hutchinson, B. (2020). Economic effects of the double burden of malnutrition. *The Lancet.* 395 (10218): 156–164.

Nnyepi, M.S., Gwisai, N., Lekgoa, M., and Seru, T. (2015). Evidence of the nutrition transition in southern Africa. *Proc. Nutr. Soc.* 74 (4): 478–486.

Ong, K.K., Ahmed, M.L., Emmett, P.M. et al. (2000). Association between postnatal catch-up growth and obesity in childhood: Prospective cohort study. *BMJ* 320 (7240): 967–971.

Pedro, T.M., Kahn, K., Pettifor, J.M. et al. (2014). Under- and overnutrition and evidence of metabolic disease risk in rural black South African children and adolescents. *S. Afr. J. Clin. Nutr.* 27 (4): 198–200.

Pomeroy, E., Stock, J.T., Stanojevic, S. et al. (2014). Stunting, adiposity, and the individual-level 'dual burden' among urban lowland and rural highland Peruvian children. *Am. J. Hum. Biol.* 26: 481–490.

Popkin, B.M. (2015). Nutrition transition and the global diabetes pandemic. *Curr. Diab. Rep.* 15 (9): 64.

Popkin, B.M. and Gordon-Larson, P. (2004). The nutrition transition: worldwide obesity dynamics and their determinants. *Int. J. Obes.* 28: S2–S9.

Ramachandran, P. (2011). Nutrition transition in India. *Bull. Nutr. Found. India* 32 (2): 1–5.

Rogero, M.M. and Calder, P.C. (2018). Obesity, inflammation, toll-like receptor 4 and fatty acids. *Nutrients* 10 (4): 432.

Sekiyama, M., Roosita, K., and Ohtsuka, R. (2017). Locally sustainable school lunch intervention improves hemoglobin and hematocrit levels and body mass index among elementary schoolchildren in rural West Java, Indonesia. *Nutrients* 9: 868.

Sharkey, J.R., Nalty, C., Johnson, C.M., and Dean, W.R. (2012, 2012). Children's very low food security is associated with increased dietary intakes in energy, fat and added sugar among Mexican-origin children (6-11y) in Texas border *Colonias*. *BMC Paediatr.* 12 (16): https://doi.org/10.1186/1471-2431-12-16.

The GBD 2015 Obesity Collaborators (2015). Health effects of overweight and obesity in 195 countries over 25 years. *N. Engl. J. Med.* 377 (1): 13–27.

Tzioumis, E. and Adair, L.S. (2014). Childhood dual burden of under- and overnutrition in low- and middle-income countries: a critical review. *Food Nutr. Bull.* 35 (2): 230–243.

Walker, S.P., Chang, S.M., Wright, A. et al. (2015). Early childhood stunting is associated with lower developmental levels in the subsequent generation of children. *J. Nutr.* 145 (4): 823–828.

Whitney, E. and Rolfes, S.R. (2019). *Understanding Nutrition*, 15e. Boston: Cengage.

WHO (2004). Appropriate body-mass index for Asian populations and its implications for policy and intervention strategies. *Lancet* 363 (9403): 157–163. https://doi.org/10.1016/S0140-6736(03)15268-3.

WHO (2017). *The double burden of malnutrition. Policy brief*. Geneva: World Health Organisation.

Wojcicki, J.M. (2014). The double burden household in sub-Saharan Africa: maternal overweight and obesity and childhood undernutrition from the year 2000: results from World Health Organisation data (WHO) and demographic health surveys. *BMC Public Health* 14: 1124.

Wolde, M., Berhan, Y., and Chala, A. (2015, 2015). Determinants of underweight, stunting and wasting among school children. *BMC Public Health* 15 (8): https://doi.org/10.1186/s12889-014-1337-2.

World Bank (2020). Urban Development. Available from : https://www.worldbank.org/en/topic/urbandevelopment/overview#1

9 Food Security, Sustainable Food and Agriculture

9.1 Introduction

Approximately 10% of the global population suffers from severe food insecurity (FAO 2018). There are approximately 60 million children who suffer from wasting and 160 million children who are stunted worldwide. Accessibility, affordability, utilisation and stability of food systems affect food security. While great progress has been made to reduce the number of malnourished children across the globe, changes to the food system such as the first green revolution have also resulted in 1.5 billion overweight adults, of which 600 million are obese. The food system is a major contributor to climate change and is affected by climate change. Some of the largest effects of climate change are already disproportionately affecting the populations at the highest risk of food insecurity. The minimally acceptable and sustainable diet is unaffordable for 1.2 billion people across the world. The UN Sustainable Development Goals (SDGs) aim to eliminate malnutrition in all its forms by 2030 through a multisectoral approach. However, many countries are not on track to meet these goals. In addition, future challenges in sustainability and feeding the human population may undermine the progress already being made to meet the SDGs. There has been recent growing interest in sustainable food systems from high-income countries that have resulted in promising innovations. However, the acceptability and appropriateness of these innovations in low- and middle-income country settings must be addressed.

9.1.1 Food Security

Food security refers to the availability of food, the ability to access food and the adequacy of available food for human health. However, food security is difficult to define as a concept (Barrett 2010). The definition of food security has evolved through time, and the main differences involve determining the adequacy of nutritional intake, whether food security refers to populations, households or individuals (Maxwell and

Nutrition and Global Health, First Edition. Shawn W. McLaren.
© 2023 John Wiley & Sons Ltd. Published 2023 by John Wiley & Sons Ltd.

Smith 1992). An early United Nations definition of food security is the 'availability at all times of adequate world supplies of basic food-stuffs to sustain a steady expansion of food consumption and to offset fluctuations in production and prices' (United Nations 1975). This definition emphasises the importance of agricultural economics in ensuring availability of food. The financial aspect of food security is seen again in the definition offered by Valdes and Konandreas (1981), which states that food security is the 'certain ability to finance needed imports to meet immediate targets for consumption levels'. However, inequality in food distribution and access can result in food insecurity on a household or individual level even if a country is considered food secure on aggregate. Insufficient access to food is one of the underlying causes of malnutrition according to the UNICEF conceptual framework (UNICEF 1990). The South African General Household Survey that took place in 2013 revealed that 79.6% of South Africans had adequate access to food, 17.6% had inadequate food access and 6.1% had severely inadequate access (Statistics South Africa 2013). The data from Statistics South Africa demonstrate the difference between aggregate food security and household food security. According to Smith et al. (2006), household-level surveys are able to improve the accuracy of estimates of national food supplies and the distribution of food energy through the population.

Jonsson and Toole (1991) defined food security as 'access to food, adequate in quality and quantity to fulfil all nutritional requirements for all household members throughout the year'.

Nutritional adequacy is an important consideration in food security. Meeting the nutritional needs of a population is difficult to define. Reutlinger (1985) offers a contrasting definition of food security by Alamgir and Arora (1991) as 'enough food available to ensure a minimum necessary intake by all members', with his earlier definition 'access by all people at all times to enough food for an active, healthy life'. The difference here is an emphasis on the promotion of health against the prevention of deficiency as the measure of adequacy.

The Jonsson and Toole (1991) definition of food security emphasises the availability of food throughout the year as an important aspect of food security. UNICEF's (1990) definition of food security is 'the assurance of food to meet needs throughout every season of the year'. Importance is placed on seasonality and availability of food in these definitions. A major cause of acute hunger and undernutrition in the developing world is the annual 'hunger season', characterised by reduced harvest stocks, high food prices and job scarcity driven by increased competition for work (Vaitla et al. 2009). Catch-up growth amongst wasted infants has been found to be slower during the hunger season (Schoenbucher et al. 2019). Season of birth is thought to influence malnutrition (stunting and wasting) risk amongst infants (Briend 2019). However, the causes of seasonal effect on malnutrition risk are not yet clear and are thought to be related to increased infectious disease risk during the hunger season or possibly due to seasonal changes in human milk oligosaccharides, which influence infant growth (Schoenbucher et al. 2019). A definition of food insecurity given by Phillips and Taylor (1990) states 'that food insecurity exists when members of a household have an inadequate diet for part or all of the year or face the possibility of an inadequate diet in the future'. This definition also alludes to seasonal variability in food security over the course of the year.

Food security is an important aspect of national economic, social and health policy. Food security concerns food availability and access. While policy makers may be concerned with population estimates of food security for planning, individual- and household-level food security is more likely to take into account the differences in distribution and resources across a population and therefore give a more accurate understanding of food security. The aim of ensuring food security can vary widely between regions, with some focusing on the prevention of deficiency and malnutrition, while others define nutritional adequacy as nutrition required for promoting health and activity. Seasonal variations in the availability of food, and therefore food security, should be taken into account when discussing food security.

The current definition of food security, adopted at the 1996 World Food Summit, is 'a situation that exists when all people, at all times, have physical, social and economic access to sufficient, safe and nutritious food that meets their dietary needs and food preferences for an active and healthy life' (World Food Summit 1996). The four components of food security are the physical availability of food, economic and physical access to food, food utilisation and the stability of these three dimensions of food security over time. These four components are all addressed by the current definition of food security.

9.2 The Dimensions of Food Security

9.2.1 Availability

The first World Food Conference which took place in 1974, focused on the problem of global production, trade and stocks. Hence, the original food security debate focused on an adequate supply of food and ensuring the stability of these supplies through food reserves.

Subsequent food security efforts focused primarily on food production and storage mechanisms to offset fluctuations in global supply and ensure the ability to import food when needed. Food availability addresses the 'supply side' of food security and is determined by the level of food production, stock levels and net trade.

9.2.2 Access

Since the early 1980s, the importance of food access was increasingly recognised as a key determinant of food security. Hence, food production is just one of several means that people have to acquire the food that they need. Concerns about insufficient food access have resulted in a greater policy focus on incomes and expenditure in achieving food security objectives. This has brought food security closer to the poverty reduction agenda.

9.2.3 Utilisation

A third dimension – food utilisation – has become increasingly prominent in food security discussions since the 1990s. Utilisation is commonly understood as the way the body makes the most of various nutrients in the food. This food security dimension is primarily determined by people's health status. Food security was traditionally perceived as consuming sufficient protein and energy (food quantity). The importance of micro-nutrients for a balanced and nutritious diet (food quality) is now well appreciated.

9.2.4 Stability

The phrase 'all people, at all times' is integral to the definition of food security and is key to achieving national food security objectives. Different people are food secure to varying degrees and will be affected by adverse events differently. People's food security situation may change. Adverse weather conditions, political instability or economic factors may impact the food security status. For food security objectives to be realised, all four dimensions must be fulfilled simultaneously. For example, even if people have money (access), if there is no food available in the market (availability), people are at risk of food insecurity. Furthermore, food security is also about quality, and that your body must be healthy to enable the nutrients to be absorbed (utilisation).

These three dimensions should be stable over time and should not be affected negatively by natural, social, economic or political factors.

9.3 Duration and Severity of Food Insecurity

The duration and severity of food insecurity affect people's lives in different ways. Inadequate food consumption may be a short-term experience or an ongoing problem. Therefore, food insecurity is often divided into two categories – transitory food insecurity and chronic food insecurity. Chronic food insecurity is often the result of poverty, lack of assets and inadequate access to productive or financial resources. Transitional food insecurity is relatively unpredictable and can occur suddenly.

Price shocks, in which food prices increase dramatically over a short period, and natural disasters such as drought, flooding and crop failure often result in transitory food insecurity (Bang et al. 2018). Transitory food insecurity elicits a response from humanitarian agencies. Chronic food insecurity is generally treated as a developmental issue (Maxwell et al. 2010). This division between chronic and transitory food insecurity is similar to the organisation of programmes in response to acute and chronic malnutrition – where wasting or acute malnutrition is again treated as the area for emergency humanitarian aid while chronic malnutrition, manifested as stunting amongst children, is addressed by developmental agencies (Angood et al. 2016). Physiological links between wasting and stunting are not yet well understood, although it is emerging that stunting may be related to repeated episodes of wasting in early infancy and childhood (Briend 2019). Similarly, food systems need to be sustainable, resilient and efficient at all times in order to achieve food and nutrition security, which implies an intersection between development and emergency planning for food security (Bilali et al. 2018).

Considering the severity of food insecurity instead of duration in characterising food security might help to select the most appropriate response (Devereux 2006). Devereux (2006) has suggested four categories of food security based on a combination of severity and duration, namely moderate chronic, severe chronic, moderate transitory and severe transitory. Moderate chronic includes moderate hunger, differentiated from severe chronic that is characterised by high infant mortality rates. Moderate transitory food insecurity refers to hungry season food insecurity, while severe transitory food insecurity refers to food crises (Devereux 2006).

Addressing extreme poverty has an impact on food security indicators (Devereux et al. 2019). A package of support that included asset transfers, training and coaching and access to savings facilities improved food security, reducing the number of months of hunger and increasing dietary diversity and meals eaten per day (Devereux et al. 2019). Importantly, the effects generated by this approach were shown to be sustained at a two-year follow-up.

Nutrient requirements are defined for individuals but measured at the household level (Schneider and Masters 2019). In a Malawian cohort, approximately one-third to two-thirds of households reach nutrient requirements. It was found that there were no significant associations between household food security and seasonality or volatility in market costs, but increased household size reduced the odds of meeting nutritional adequacy (Schneider and Masters 2019), meaning that intra-household distribution of food and resources is an important factor in food security and nutritionally adequate intakes.

9.4 Vulnerability to Food Insecurity

Prior to the modern industrial food system and global transportation of agricultural products, famines were often experienced locally. When food supplies were reduced by natural disaster, conflict and political or economic turmoil, the demand for food supplies raised prices, further worsening the prevalence of starvation.

By the middle of the twentieth century, improvements in international transportation had resulted in a shift from local to world food prices for basic commodities. This in turn lowered the possibility of famines in all regions except for those with the least developed transportation infrastructure. As local food prices are now largely reflective of international food prices, in a system of free exchange, the risk of greatly increased food prices in famine-struck regions is lowered. However, even as transportation systems are improved, the problem of distribution is affected by other factors, including import and export tariffs, quota systems and cartel agreements (Keys et al. 1950).

A major determinant of resource allocation is pricing. Prices that consumers pay for food products are influenced by disturbances in production or supply chains. Important factors that result in food insecurity are natural disasters, conflict and political instability and hyperinflation (FAO 2018). While these factors are responsible for poor household food security in affected regions of the world, national policies can help to protect consumers against volatile international markets (FAO 2018).

Food security and dietary diversity are significantly higher in urban locations than peri-urban and rural ones (Chakona and Shackleton 2017b). Peri-urban settlements are at the highest risk of food insecurity resulting from higher levels of unemployment and poverty in combination with a lack of access to land (Chakona and Shackleton 2017b). In rural areas where subsistence agriculture takes place, there is a reduced dependence on food purchasing for food security. Additionally, surplus food grown can be sold and wild foods can be collected, increasing the level of dietary diversity in rural areas (Chakona and Shackleton 2017b). Seasonal food security fluctuates throughout the year for seasonal farm workers. Food security is highest during the summer harvest and is lowest in winter (Devereux and Tavener-Smith 2019). This implies that while rural groups may have some protection against food insecurity through access to subsistence farming, they are not unaffected by food security. Furthermore, it is worth noting that dietary monotony is not related to a lack of knowledge about dietary diversity but is related to access to food and food security (Chakona and Shackleton 2017a).

Vulnerability analysis is an analytical concept developed to address the future incidence of food insecurity (Scaramozzino 2006).

Water insecurity is positively related to food insecurity (Brewis et al. 2019). Poorer water quality and increased time and labour required for collecting water impact are independently associated with worsening food security (Brewis et al. 2019). Household food security is affected by water insecurity due to the need to purchase water, which affects the household food budget (Subbaraman et al. 2015). This effect is compounded by the substantial time expenditure and opportunity costs that impact employment (Subbaraman et al. 2015). Water is required for subsistence and smallholder farming, and the availability of water for people relying on this method of food production for some or all of the year has a large impact on crop yields (Sinyolo et al. 2014). However, the contribution of subsistence farming to food security in South Africa may be small, as up to 90% of food consumed is bought at supermarkets, in both urban and rural communities (Baiphethi and Jacobs 2009). Scarcity of water can affect food preparation. Staple foods such as beans and maize porridges require a large amount of water to cook (Workman and Ureksoy 2017). Beans in particular have a high tannin content; protein and starch need to be hydrolysed for digestibility, and palatability, which requires prolonged cooking times (Elia et al. 1997). While there is a lack of empirical evidence to link cooking fuel choice to food insecurity in the same manner as water security (Sola et al. 2016), Agea et al. (2010) report that women can spend as much as four to six hours a day in collecting firewood for cooking fuel. This may infer that fuel use for cooking has a similar impact on opportunity cost and household income as water scarcity. However, the issue of cooking fuel choice is complex, and solid fuel or wood for cooking remains the most common fuel choice in many sub-Saharan African communities and is not affected by increased income (Kirimu 2015).

Food insecurity also affects developed countries, and its increase in European countries is thought to be related to a recent recession in Europe as well as unemployment, debt and housing arrears (Loopstra et al. 2015).

9.5 Global Challenges and Strategies for Food Security

Approximately half of the world's population lives in urban environments, and the proportion of people living in towns and cities is expected to increase to 70% by 2050 (United Nations 2007). The growing human population and consequent competition for land, water and energy for food production is a major challenge for food security in the twenty-first century. Overfishing, growing cities and urban areas encroaching into fertile zones and climate change are additional challenges unique to this century (Godray et al. 2010). Gu et al. (2019) have suggested four ways in which food security might be improved for rapidly growing cities. They suggest reducing food waste, combining pockets of rural land, improving farming practices and reducing meat consumption to improve food security.

The FAO (2018) definition of food waste includes any foods that were intended for human consumption but have been lost degraded or consumed by pests. Food, which is diverted away from human consumption to feed livestock, is also sometimes considered as food waste, including feeding edible by-products of food production to animals.

Current global losses and food waste are difficult to quantify; however, some estimate that up to half of all food produced is lost before it reaches the consumer (Parfitt et al. 2010). Post-harvest losses are related to technology available in a given country. Post-harvest and supply chain technology is more developed in industrialised countries and urbanised countries. The application of these technologies ranges from rudimentary post-harvest infrastructure to packing houses and storage facilities in more transitional countries and advanced cold-chain systems in industrialised countries (Parfitt et al. 2010). As post-harvest technology improves, the level of dietary diversity increases (Parfitt et al. 2010). This can be seen in the increase of the use of very perishable foods in more urban and affluent areas, and higher consumption of less perishable foods such as root vegetables and dried staple crops in less developed places. However, these perishable foods are more likely to be wasted than non-perishable. Some cities have begun collecting discarded food in separate containers, which can be converted to animal feed, reducing the amount of overall food waste by preventing food for human consumption from being diverted to animal feed. Vegetable waste in particular has great potential for animal feed use (Martin and Zufia 2016). However, in this case, it is by-products from agricultural vegetable and plant production which is diverted for animal use (Martin and Zufia 2016). Previous research has indicated that restaurant and household food waste is too high in heavy metals for safe use in animal feed production (Garcia et al. 2005). The researchers had to remove non-biodegradable waste themselves, particularly from household waste samples.

9.6 Sustainability and Agriculture

Thomas Robert Malthus developed a theory regarding population growth and population pressure – dealing specifically with food supply – in the early nineteenth century in England. In Malthus' model, population growth is checked by the availability of food. In his predictions, where population growth is exponential but food production increases in a linear fashion, the English population would reach approximately 150 million people by 1930, with 100 million of them facing starvation, unless population growth was checked by some other factor. The solutions offered by Malthus were to reduce the rate of population growth by maintaining wages at a subsistence level and to control birth rates through enforcing Victorian-era morality regarding sex. While these solutions would not be considered acceptable by today's standards, the philosophy was influential, and iterations of Malthus' model have been used to explain food security for populations.

9.7 Per capita food availability, predictions of carry capacity and population size

The rate of growth of the global human population has been declining; however, the world population doubled during the course of the twentieth century. This rapid increase was made possible by greatly increased life expectancy across the world, as a result of technological improvements in food production and medical care. However, improvements in overall agricultural production are not necessarily beneficial for the world's most vulnerable populations.

Over 1 billion people are involved in agriculture, of whom 300 million are employees in the agricultural sector. A large proportion of people working in the agricultural sector are casual or temporary workers or seasonal labourers (ILO 2014). The contribution of the world's workforce from agriculture declined by 14 to 31% between 1991 and 2013 (ILO 2014). The changing nature of agricultural work, with increased automation, means that job security is uncertain for millions of workers, with those involved in small-scale farming at a particularly high risk of interruptions to food security (ILO 2014). In addition, deforestation and depletion of soil quality threaten the sustainability of the current agricultural system.

Malthus' model was adapted during the twentieth century by the FAO (Figure 9.1). The revised model now included economic and political

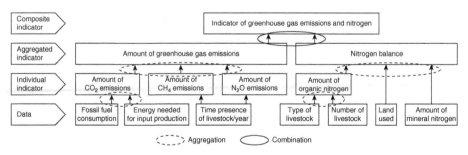

Figure 9.1: Framework of indicators for agricultural sustainability (Latruffe et al. 2016).

influences. More recent imaginations of the model include sustainability as a factor, incorporating the impact on the environment as well as environmental carrying capacity. The physical limitation of available arable land and the production of greenhouse gases are now considered in the model of food system carrying capacity for the human population.

Given these models, an important question to answer is how we will continue to feed the human population in the twenty-first century. By the mid-twentieth century, if food produced worldwide was distributed perfectly, everyone would have had enough to eat to prevent death from starvation but not enough of sufficient nutritional quality to ensure optimal nutritional status (Keys et al. 1950). This important observation raises many questions around twenty-first century predictions.

The future of the global food supply is further complicated by advancing technologies in animal feed production and biofuel production. The majority of crop production is currently comprised of cereals for human consumption such as wheat and rice. However, more than half of the population lives in urban environments (FAO 2018), and as prosperity increases, diets become more varied and higher in animal products, and less reliant on staple crops. Coarse grains and oilseeds are taking the place of staple crop production in order to be used as animal feed and for biofuel production (FAO 2018). Increasing demand for biofuels in developed countries has had the effect of increasing the prices of staple food crops. According to Renzaho et al. (2017), the current impact of increased production of crops for biofuels on climate change is not clear. As with any agricultural practice, producing crops requires land which that could potentially result in continued deforestation, as well as other inputs such as fossil fuels. The unknown impact of competition between biofuel production demand and staple food crop demand led these researchers to suggest that agendas around biofuel production should protect rural communities from food insecurity as an unintended consequence of this competition (Renzaho et al. 2017).

These current and future conditions in agricultural systems will have an impact on global aims to reduce poverty and eradicate hunger, as outlined in the SDGs. Strategies to prevent household food insecurity may include biofortification of staple crops to ensure better nutritional composition and help to ensure that staples are adequate to meet nutritional requirements. Strategies should focus on encouraging sustainable agricultural practices, considering both the need to improve food security for a growing population as well as reducing contributions to climate change. There may be a role to play for improved nutrition education, in order to improve dietary diversity and micronutrient adequacy.

9.8 Growing a Vitamin A Garden

Growing a vitamin A garden is a food-based approach to improving micronutrient status. Resources are required in order for a vitamin A garden to be successful. First, gardeners will need access to land to grow their food. It has been suggested that a garden sized $100\,m^2$ can support a family and produce enough surplus crops to sell, give to neighbours or donate to education centres. Initial costs required for starting a vegetable garden can be inhibitive. Money will be needed for soil, compost, mulch, seeds and seedlings and gardening tools such as spades, garden forks and watering cans. It is a good idea to fence off a garden, as this helps to prevent theft and keeps livestock out of the garden. The fence is an additional expense. In many regions, there are schemes that aim to assist communities and families to overcome the initial costs of starting a garden. Support is also available in the form of knowledge transfer training schemes to assist with starting and maintaining a vegetable garden. People should be at the centre of planning for vegetable gardens as this is a strong determinant of the success of the vegetable garden. Domestic gardens are managed by households. Here, motivation may be driven by livelihood and additional income from the garden produce. In community gardens, income generation can be a strong motivator. School gardens tend to benefit from dedicated gardeners, such as a school maintenance person, instead of teachers. Maintaining vegetable gardens requires continuous access to seeds and seedlings. In order for vegetable gardens to generate income, they should have access to markets. These may be formal or informal. Foods high in vitamin A include pumpkin and squashes and spinach and carrots.

MASHED PUMPKIN WITH PEANUT BUTTER

Ingredients

One medium pumpkin or bitter melon, peeled, seeded and cut into cubes
Water
Three cups maize meal
One and a half cups peanuts or three tablespoons peanut butter
Half teaspoon salt
Sugar to taste (for bitter melon)

1. Boil pumpkin or bitter melon in salted water until soft.
2. Mash until smooth and liquid.
3. Add maize meal and cook for 30 minutes, stirring occasionally.
4. Add peanuts or peanut butter and salt.

References

Agea, J.G., Kirangwa, D., Waiswa, D., and Okia, C.A. (2010). Household firewood consumption in Kalisizo sub-country, Central Uganda. *Ethnobot. Leaflets* 14: 841–855.

Alamgir, M. and Arora, P. (1991). Providing Food Security for all. In: *International Fund for Agricultural Development*. USA: New York University Press.

Angood, C., Khara, T., Dolan, C. et al. (2016). Research priorities on the relationship between wasting and stunting. *PLoS One* 11 (5): e0153221.

Baiphethi, M.N. and Jacobs, P.T. (2009). The contribution of subsistence farming to food security in South Africa. *Agric. Econ. Res. Policy Pract. Southern Africa* 48 (4): 459–482.

Bang, H.N., Miles, L., and Gordon, R. (2018). Enhancing local livelihoods resilience and food security in the face of frequent flooding in Africa: a disaster management perspective. *J. Afr. Stud. Dev.* 10 (7): 85–100.

Barrett, C.V. (2010). Measuring food insecurity. *Science* 327 (5967): 825–828.

Bilali, H.E., Callenius, C., Strassner, C., and Probst, L. (2018). Food and nutrition security and sustainability transitions in food systems. *Food Energy Security* 8 (2): e00154.

Brewis, A., Workman, C., Wutich, A. et al. (2019). Household water insecurity is strongly associated with food insecurity: evidence from 27 sites in low- and middle-income countries. *Am. J. Hum. Biol.* 31 (2): e23309.

Briend, A. (2019). The complex relationship between wasting and stunting. *Am. J. Clin. Nutr.* 110 (2): 271–272.

Chakona, G. and Shackleton, C.M. (2017a). Voices of the hungry: a qualitative measure of household food access and food insecurity in South Africa. *Agric. Food Secur.* (6): 66.

Chakona, G. and Shackleton, C. (2017b). Minimum dietary diversity scores for women indicate micronutrient adequacy and food insecurity status in South African towns. *Nutrients* 9: 812.

Devereux S (2006). Distinguishing between chronic and transitory food insecurity in emergency needs assessments. SENAC, World Food Programme, Rome.

Devereux, S. and Tavener-Smith, L. (2019). Seasonal food insecurity among farm workers in the Northern Cape, South Africa. *Nutrients* 11 (7): 1535.

Devereux, S., Roelen, K., Sabates, R. et al. (2019). Graduating from food insecurity: evidence from graduation projects in Burundi and Rwanda. *Food Secur.* 11 (1): 219–232.

Elia, F.M., Hosfield, G.L., Kelly, J.D., and Uebersax, M.A. (1997). Genetic analysis and interrelationships between traits for cooking time, water absorption, and protein and tannin content of Andean dry beans. *Journal of the American Society for Horticultural Science* 122 (4): 512–518.

FAO (2018). *World Food and Agriculture – Statistical Pocket Book 2018*. Rome: Food and Agriculture Organisation of the United Nations.

Garcia, A.J., Esteban, M.B., Marquez, M.C., and Ramos, P. (2005). Biodegradable municipal solid waste: characterisation and potential use as animal foodstuffs. *Waste Manage. (Oxford)* 25: 780–787.

Godray, H.C.J., Beddington, J.R., Crute, I.R. et al. (2010). Food security: the challenge of feeding 9 billion people. *Science* 327 (5967): 812–818.

Gu, B., Zhang, X., Bai, X. et al. (2019). Four steps to food security for swelling cities. *Nature* 566: 31–33.

ILO (2014). *Key Indicators of the Labour Market*. Geneva: International Labour Organisation.

Jonsson, U. and Toole, D. (1991). *Household Food Security and Nutrition: A Conceptual Analysis*. New York: UNICEF.

Keys, A., Brozek, J., Henschel, A. et al. (1950). *The Biology of Human Starvation*, vol. 1. Minneapolis: The University of Minnesota Press.

Kirimu, A. (2015). Cooking fuel preferences among Ghanaian households: an empirical analysis. *Energy Sustain. Dev.* 207: 10–17.

Latruffe, L., Diazabakana, A., Bockstaller, C. et al. (2016). Measurement of sustainability in agriculture: a review of indicators. *Stud. Agric. Econ.* 118 (3): 123–130. ISSN 2063- 047.

Loopstra, R., Reeves, A., and Stuckler, D. (2015). Rising food insecurity in Europe. *Lancet* 385 (9982): 2041.

Martin, D.S. and Zufia, S.R.J. (2016). Valorisation of food waste to produce new raw materials for animal feed. *Food Chem.* 198 (1): 68–74.

Maxwell, S. and Smith, M. (1992). *Household Food Security: A Conceptual Review*. New York: UNICEF.

Maxwell, D., Webb, P., Coates, J., and Wirth, J. (2010). Fit for purpose? Rethinking food security responses in protracted humanitarian crises. *Food Policy* 35: 91–97.

Parfitt, J., Barthel, M., and MacNaughton, S. (2010). Food waste within food supply chains: quantification and potential to change to 2050. *Philos. Trans. R. Soc.* 365: 3065–3081.

Phillips, T. and Taylor, D. (1990). Optimal control of food insecurity: a conceptual framework. *Am. J. Agric. Econ.* 72 (5): 1304–1310.

Renzaho, A.M.N., Kamara, J.K., and Toole, M. (2017). Biofuel production and its impact on food security in low and middle income countries: implications for the post-2015 sustainable development goals. *Renewable Sustainable Energy Rev.* 78: 503–516.

Reutlinger (1985). Policy options for food security. Discussion Paper Report No ARU44. Agriculture and Rural Development Department, Research Unit, World Bank, Washington DC.

Scaramozzino, P. (2006). Measuring vulnerability to food insecurity. ESA Working Paper no 06–12. Rome: FAO.

Schneider, K. and Masters, W. (2019). Nutrient adequacy at the household level and the cost of nutritious diets in Malawi. *Curr. Dev. Nutr.* 3 (31): 816.

Schoenbucher, S.M., Dolan, C., Mwangome, M. et al. (2019). The relationship between stunting and wasting: a retrospective cohort analysis of longitudinal data in Gambian children from 1976 to 2016. *Am. J. Clin. Nutr.* 110 (2): 498–507.

Sinyolo, S., Mudhara, M., and Wale, E. (2014). The impact of smallholder irrigation on household welfare: the case of Tugela Ferry irrigation scheme in KwaZulu-Natal, South Africa. *Water SA* 40 (1): 145–156.

Smith, L.C., Alderman, H., and Aduayom, D. (2006). *Food Insecurity in Sub-Saharan Africa: New Estimates from Household Expenditure Surveys*. Washington DC: International Food Policy Research Institute.

Sola, P., Ochieng, C., Yila, J., and Liyama, M. (2016). Links between energy access and food security in sub-Saharan Africa: an exploratory review. *Food Security* 8 (3): 635–642.

Statistics South Africa (2013). *General Household Survey 2013*. Pretoria: Statistics South Africa.

Subbaraman, R., Nolan, L., Sawant, K. et al. (2015). Multidimensional measurement of household water poverty in a Mumbai slum: looking beyond water quality. *PLoS One* 10 (7): e0133241.

United Nations (1975). Report of the World Food Conference, Rome, 5-16 November 1974. New York: United Nations.

United Nations (2007). World urbanization prospects. The 2007 revision population database.

United Nations Children's Fund (UNICEF) (1990). UNICEF Conceptual Framework. https://www.unicef.org/nutrition/training/2.5/4.html.

Vaitla, B., Devereux, S., and Swan, S.H. (2009). Seasonal hunger: a neglected problem with proven solutions. *PLoS Med.* 6 (6): e1000101.

Valdes, A. and Konandreas, P. (1981). Assessing food insecurity based on national aggregates in developing countries. In: *Food Security for Developing Countries* (ed. A. Valdes). Boulder: Westview Press.

Workman, C.L. and Ureksoy, H. (2017). Water insecurity in syndemic context: understanding the psycho-environmental stress of water insecurity in Lesotho, Africa. *Social Sci. Med.* 179: 52–60.

World Food Summit (1996). Rome Declaration on World Food Security.

10 Working in the Global Health Environment

10.1 Introduction

The scope of the global health professional is broad. Health workers in this field may spend their time studying epidemics and their treatment and prevention. Some of the most important challenges in global health today include treating and preventing infectious diseases such as human immunodeficiency virus, tuberculosis and malaria. In the field of global health, workers may be involved in investigating vaccine coverage, the effects of behaviours on public health outcomes or reducing inequities in access to health systems. This may be achieved through monitoring and evaluating a community's healthcare system to identify areas for improvement or predict potential problems. At this larger scale, those working in global health work alongside national leaders, governmental agencies, relief organisations and non-governmental organisations (NGOs) to bring about improved health outcomes for populations. They help to develop policies, procedures and plans to improve health. On a more local scale, global health workers work with communities to identify barriers to improved health, identify at-risk groups in the community, provide training and education on health issues and support improvements in health infrastructure. As we have seen in previous chapters, nutrition, disease and access to health are intimately related. Nutrition is an important aspect of development and implementing nutrition-specific and nutrition-sensitive interventions in areas of global health concern such as maternal and child health, and infectious diseases and humanitarian emergencies will have a direct impact.

The key focus of global health work is conducting data-driven research and educational outreach. The topics explored in this chapter include planning interventions, deciding how interventions will be monitored and evaluated, accessing resources, including funding as well as community mobilisation. Of crucial importance is the topic of ethics in global health. When interventions are designed and implemented, target populations need to be directly involved.

Nutrition and Global Health, First Edition. Shawn W. McLaren.
© 2023 John Wiley & Sons Ltd. Published 2023 by John Wiley & Sons Ltd.

10.2 Planning a Programme

This section describes the reasons for programme planning and the steps that should be taken in the planning process. It incorporates monitoring and evaluation in the planning process. Planning clarifies what the programme aims to achieve, which aims take priority and how the programme will achieve its aims. Existing frameworks for planning interventions include intervention mapping (Figure 10.1) (Bartholomew et al. 1998), the conceptual framework for planning intervention-related research (de Zoysa et al. 1998; Figure 10.2), the PRECEDE-PROCEED model (Figure 10.3) (Green and Kreuter 2005), the framework for design evaluation of complex interventions to improve health (Campbell et al. 2007), Medical Research Council (MRC) guidance for the development and evaluation of complex interventions (MRC 2008) and the design for behaviour changes framework (CORE Group 2008).

Each of these models or frameworks has elements in common. Each model begins by identifying the problem faced by a community. Outcomes that the intervention aims to achieve are then defined. Ongoing monitoring and evaluation informs implementation at each step of the intervention. The essence of each of these models can be found in the following six steps to design a quality intervention:

1. Defining and understanding the problem and its causes
2. Identifying which causal or contextual factors are modifiable: which have the greatest scope for change and who would benefit the most
3. Deciding on the mechanisms of change

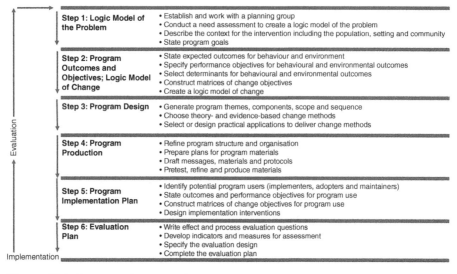

Figure 10.1: Intervention mapping.

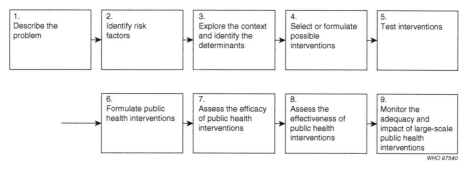

Figure 10.2: Conceptual framework for planning intervention-based research (De Zoysa et al. 1998).

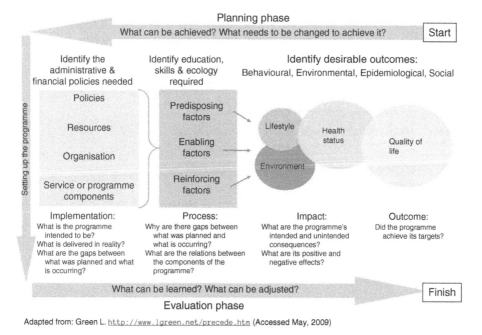

Figure 10.3: PREDE-PROCEED model.

Source: Adapted from Green and Kreuter 2005.

4. Clarify how these will be delivered
5. Testing and adapting the intervention
6. Collecting sufficient evidence of effectiveness to proceed to a rigorous intervention (Wight et al. 2016)

When defining and understanding the problem and its causes, it is useful to identify a nutrition-specific or nutrition-sensitive area, topic or issue. Once this has been identified, it is then a useful step to identify causal and contextual factors that are modifiable. These factors can be ranked based on their scope for change and potential beneficiaries. Then, the next step is to decide on how change can be achieved.

Once the problem has been explored in depth, a framework can be selected which will guide the intervention. Health workers could identify conceptual frameworks that are relevant to the current situation, make use of published evidence, projects carried out in the past which were successful, and established interventions in the area.

To clarify how the intervention will be delivered, health workers should develop a clear aim of the project. The scope of the project should be defined. Considerations to make include the feasibility of the intervention, the time frame, resources available, funding available and specific needs of the target group or beneficiaries. For an intervention to be successful, the values of the stakeholders and the organisation carry out the intervention. The values of the funding organisation are also likely to influence decisions. They will need to identify what is achievable.

One of the first steps in implementing an intervention will usually be applying for funding for the intervention. This requires careful planning – funders will want to provide resources to projects that are likely to deliver on their promises. Careful planning can help build funders' confidence in the intervention they are proposing.

Steps in the planning process are as follows:

1. Analyse opportunities and constraints
2. SWOT analysis
3. Determine objectives and develop a plan to achieve them
4. 'Logframe' analysis
5. Determine verifiable indicators
6. Assess existing capacity and potential
7. Planning for long-term community-based therapeutic care (CTC) programming
8. Determine resource requirements
9. Use a planning feedback loop

10.3 Assessing Community Capacity and Resource Requirements

This section discusses identifying key community figures, groups and organisations, as well as formal and informal routes of communication, and explores motivation to change. It outlines the concepts of institutional frameworks, funding and supplies and expertise.

Interventions are more likely to be successful if the target population is part of the solution. Identifying key community figures can be an important part of incorporating community structures into an intervention. If leaders already recognised by the community are involved in the intervention, the intervention is more likely to be accepted by the community. It is also useful to establish links with community groups and organisations that already exist in the community. The intervention can make use of pre-existing social infrastructure to address new problems. Local agricultural groups, women's groups, youth centres, infant and young child feeding groups, and co-ops set up by previous government interventions can help. In any community, there are formal and informal channels of communication. Identifying these and making effective use of them can assist in improving recruitment into the intervention, communicate successes and identify needs of the community. In this way, community motivating factors can be identified and used to improve the effectiveness of the intervention. Alongside pre-existing social infrastructure, the intervention can make use of pre-existing health and care structures. Local pathways for disease treatment or social support, for example, may be used in the intervention as part of service delivery. If these structures are strong, they can provide a vehicle for reaching beneficiaries, and if the community identifies problems with these structures, the intervention may work to improve these. These steps may be informal processes. Combining interventions with pre-existing institutional frameworks such as local and national health and social care departments can provide support in the forms of finance, human resources and knowledge or experience. Building on pre-existing social structures will help to improve the sustainability of a project – once the funding terms ends, the ideal situation is that the work is continued by the community itself. Therefore, mobilising communities is valuable to the long-term success of interventions.

10.3.1 Funding and Supplies

Donor agencies are crucial for intervention success. Donor agencies can be categorised into two major groups – those providing funds for emergency relief programmes and those providing financial support for development programmes.

10.3.2 Expertise (Knowledge and Skills)

One of the greatest financial commitments for an intervention is staff. During the planning stages, the need for salaried staff and local volunteer workers needs to be addressed. Salaried staff may include project managers, clinicians, facilitators, administrative and support staff, statisticians and project evaluators. Local volunteer workers may work without pay or may be provided with a stipend or other incentives for their services. Knowledge transfer and ongoing training are important for both salaried staff and local volunteers. Ensuring that knowledge transfer takes place – providing the skills and training necessary to allow volunteer workers and community workers to carry out the intervention – is crucial for sustainability of projects and interventions.

10.3.3 Monitoring and Evaluation

Monitoring and evaluation takes place throughout an intervention. It allows planners to determine whether the project is on track to meet its aims for delivery and implementation and ensures funders that their investment is being used appropriately. Monitoring and evaluation will often make use of periodic reports to assess the successes and failures of interventions. Where successes are identified, steps can be taken to consolidate these. Where failures to deliver or bottlenecks in programmes are identified, appropriate steps can be taken to resume programme efficiency.

Key question	Tools	Data
Delivering on commitments	Trends Simple correlations	National surveys Expert opinion surveys
Effectiveness of interventions	Econometric models Participatory approaches	National surveys Targeted surveys Expert opinion surveys
Consistency with initial targets	Simulation models Participatory approaches	Assessment of effectiveness Expert opinion surveys
Exploring better interventions	Simulation models Participatory approaches	Assessment of effectiveness and consistency

10.4 Community Mobilisation

This section discusses project ownership and sustainability, community sensitisation, case finding and follow-up pathways.

Including the community as active members of an intervention comes with many advantages. Chiefly, it improves coverage and encourages community ownership of the project and therefore results in greater chances of sustainability. Community sensitisation helps to increase active participation in interventions. The purpose of community sensitisation is to inform the local community of the plans for the intervention and to get the community to become actively involved in the programme. This may take the form of informal conversations with local leadership – village leaders, traditional healers and leadership, elders in the community, church leaders and head clinicians. Training sessions with community workers and volunteers are useful platforms for communicating the needs of the community and aims of the intervention. Community members can also be made aware of scheduled activities related to the intervention through formal and informal channels of communication.

Community health workers (CHWs) are employed in many low- and middle-income countries as part of the health system. They have been used to address the shortage of skilled health workers in these countries (Lehmann and Sanders 2007). CHWs are community members who provide basic health services within their own communities (Lehmann and Sanders 2007).

CHWs can play roles in interventions. They may assist with case finding. As community members themselves, they will be aware of at-risk members of the community, as well as the local challenges faced by the community in terms of access to services and service delivery. Therefore, they can make valuable contributions to intervention projects through their local knowledge and provide insights into the best approaches that can be taken in their specific context. Their familiarity with local community members can help to foster trust with the intervention organisation.

Case finding activities may be facilitated with the help of CHWs. In many instances, there is a mixture of self-referral and active case finding which takes place as part of routine health services. CHWs may be involved in setting up awareness or screening activities, making use of local infrastructure and community centres such as creches, churches, health post mobile clinics and clinics to provide decentralised services to communities. CHWs can play roles in follow-up with identified cases. They can help to identify problems and support continued community sensitisation.

10.4.1 Population Behaviour Change

Designing interventions and working in public health nutrition relies on changing population behaviours to elicit more desirable health outcomes. Key roles in influencing population health behaviours are played by governments and NGOs. Governments establish regulatory frameworks and influence nutrition and health behaviour by regulating food and pharmaceutical industries, enforcing laws and developing action plans. Governments are responsible for developing and implementing policy frameworks, surveillance activities, funding research and coordinating different sectors in the economy to address specific challenges. Governments are often responsible for health services. NGOs play a role in building community capacity, empowering people at a grassroots level and influencing policy. NGOs may also fund research. These two groups, governments and NGOs, draw on existing strategies for behaviour change in order to bring about positive changes in health and nutrition outcomes.

Behaviour change in individuals may rely on individual motivation and circumstances. Excessive alcohol consumption, drug and tobacco use, and excessive salt and fat intakes are considered undesirable health behaviours that lead to negative health outcomes. The aim of public health interventions is to shift behaviours towards more desirable ones, such as eating plenty of vegetables and fruit, exercising regularly, avoiding excessive alcohol consumption and therefore improving health outcomes amongst populations such as mortality risk, life expectancy, heart disease and cancer risk. Influencing behaviour can be made more effective by understanding motivation for behaviours and directing behaviours towards desirable outcomes.

10.4.2 Understanding Motivation

Motivation is a collection of brain processes that direct behaviours and is not limited to choices and pursuing goals. In reality, motivation also includes drives, habits, desires, instincts and self-regulation. Public health intervention models that rely purely on health messages and communication are often ineffective as they do not address underlying mechanisms that explain behaviour. Contextual factors such as the built environment, access to resources, access to basic services, education and health systems, and poverty and social class are all factors that influence behaviour. The COM-B model can be used to analyse behaviour in context (Figure 10.4).

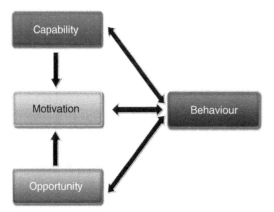

Figure 10.4: COM-B system for analysing behaviour in context.

The COM-B model assumes that capability, motivation and opportunity all need to be present before a behaviour can occur and interact as part of a system (similar in a sense to the 'triangle of fire' – for a fire to start, an ignition source, fuel and oxygen are all required at the same time; without one of these elements, the fire goes out or does not start). Motivation for a target behaviour, such as exercising 30 minutes a day or eating more vegetables and fruit, must be stronger than other competing behaviours in order for the desired behaviour to take place. It is important to remember that motivation includes habit and instinct, and so many behaviours can be difficult to overcome consciously. Motivation may be reflective, or it may be automatic. Reflective motivation refers to conscious decisions an individual makes to reach a desirable goal. Automatic motivation refers to unconscious decisions made almost as though by reflex, such as smoking when stressed or overeating when hungry. An individual must be capable of a given behaviour in order to act out the behaviour. The opportunity to act out a specific behaviour must also be present for a behaviour to occur. The opportunity can be social, or it could be environmental. Social opportunity may be embedded in culture and deems certain behaviours acceptable and others not. Environmental opportunity is an important aspect of public health. If a population is unable to access or afford healthy food and an adequate diet, no amount of motivational change will elicit a change in behaviour.

The benefit of using a comprehensive approach to eliciting behaviour change is that it addresses the combination of factors that lead to an undesirable behaviour. At a population health level, considering motivation for behaviour results in a fuller range of options for interventions being considered. It results in analysing behaviour in the context in which it takes place and accounts for environmental changes that may need to occur in order to elicit behavioural change.

Capability can be augmented through education and training – providing people with the opportunity to become capable of a particular behaviour (Figure 10.5). This may be important in breastfeeding, for example where specific skills are taught to new mothers to breastfeed their

Capability	Motivation	Opportunity
Educate	Expose to	Offer
Train	Inform	Provide
Help	Discuss	Prompt
	Suggest	Constrain
	Encourage	
	Incentivise	
	Ask	
	Order	
	Plead	
	Coerce	
	Force	

Figure 10.5: Behaviours associated with the COM-B model.

infants effectively. Motivation is more complex but can be addressed through incentive, coercion or encouragement amongst other approaches. Opportunities for desirable behaviours can be created by offering or prompting certain behaviours, while poor health behaviours can be prevented by constraining the opportunities for these behaviours (Figure 10.6). This is used in MBFI-accredited health centres, where the use of teats and pacifiers is actively discouraged or not allowed altogether.

These aspects of human behaviour can be affected by governments and NGOs.

Identifying areas for change in terms of capability, opportunity and motivation can be used to design effective behaviour change interventions (Figure 10.7). Interventions may be fiscal, in the form of taxes such as those levied to the sugar-sweetened beverage industry, and they may be

---

- **Education** Increasing knowledge or understanding

- **Persuasion** Using communication to induce positive or negative feelings or stimulate action

- **Incentivisation** Creating expectation of reward

- **Coercion** Creating expectation of punishment or cost

- **Training** Imparting skills

- **Restriction** Using rules to reduce the opportunity to engage in the target behaviour (or to increase the target behaviour by reducing the opportunity to engage in competing behaviours)

- **Environmental restructuring** Changing the physical or social context

- **Modelling** Providing an example for people to aspire to or imitate

- **Enablement** Increasing means/reducing barriers to increase capability or opportunity

---

Figure 10.6: Designing interventions based on the COM-B model.

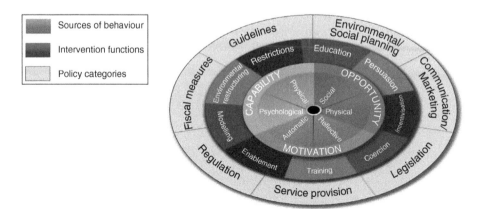

Figure 10.7: Interventions based on the COM-B model.

regulatory, such as food standards applied to hospitals, schools and food retailers. Strategies may take the form of environmental restructuring, such as improving access to health services or creating an environment conducive to physical activity.

10.5 Ethics in Global Health

This section discusses ethics in decision-making in global health interventions.

The history of public health interventions is littered with examples of misuse of power. Public health legislation such as the Epidemic Diseases Act introduced in India in 1897 allowed authorities to segregate communities and destroy infrastructure that was considered 'infected' (Loewenson et al. 2021). Not all ethical failures of public health interventions are as dramatic and obvious as this example. The World Health Organisation attempted to eradicate malaria, amongst the deadliest diseases affecting humans, through endorsing use of dichlorodiphenyltrichloroethane (DDT) to kill mosquitoes during the mid-twentieth century (Brown et al. 2006). As pointed out by Matteson (1999) in a scientific letter to *Emerging Infectious Diseases*, DDT use has been associated with undesirable birth outcomes such as low birthweight and reduced lactation. Therefore, substantial gains in managing one form of disease were made but at the expense of the health of others and of the environment.

10.5.1 Principles of Medical Ethics

There are the following four fundamental ethical principles that apply to healthcare (Beauchamp and Childress 2008):

1. Principle of **respect** for **autonomy**
2. Principle of **nonmaleficence**
3. Principle of **beneficence**
4. Principle of **justice**

Bell (2008) identified a set of principles that intersect human rights concerns and research ethics. These principles include respect for human dignity, informed consent, individual autonomy, equality, privacy and confidentiality, freedom of expression, access to information and justice. The philosophies of non-maleficence and benevolence need to direct and underpin the intentions and actions of global health work. All procedures should adhere to the ethical principles detailed by the Declaration of Helsinki (World Medical Association 2013). The principles of Autonomy, Non-maleficence, Beneficence and Justice are outlined as follows.

10.5.1.1 Autonomy

Participation in interventions must be voluntary. Where possible, participants must be asked whether they agreed to participate. With interventions concerning infants and young children, however, participants may not yet have the cognitive development required for understanding the implications of participating in scientific research. Where infants and children become upset from the procedures, health workers should not force the infant or child to participate. No community members should be forced to take part in an intervention, and no hidden data collection should take place. The right of community members to withdraw from the intervention should be clearly explained to them before they are included in the intervention. All names must be kept confidential, and participants' confidentiality should be protected.

10.5.1.2 Non-Maleficence

Methods should be employed to ensure that participant anonymity is protected. Participants' names should not be included in data collection or exported in data collection tools, and no personal identifying information should be recorded. Participants should not be harmed by the publication of the findings of an intervention.

10.5.1.3 Beneficence

The aims of the intervention should be explained to participants. The results of the intervention should be reported to the relevant health authority as well as other stakeholders, including the community.

10.5.1.4 Justice

The human rights of each participant must be respected through all stages of an intervention.

All seen at health service centres where research or interventions are taking place should be given equal and non-discriminatory access to the full spectrum of services offered at these sites, and no one must be excluded from health services rendered should they chose not to participate in research. Participants screened for nutritional problems as part of the research or intervention protocol must be referred for the appropriate intervention according to national and provincial health department policies when required. Feedback on the nutritional status of the study participant should be given to the caregiver of the participant or to the participant themselves immediately upon completion and interpretation of the measurements. Interpretation of nutritional status and appropriate nutritional interventions should be carried out as required.

An additional dimension of the ethical principle of justice is the principle of distributive justice, which refers to fairly distributing both the benefits and burdens of a public health intervention. A well-designed intervention will inevitably have a benefit to the target population at its core, such as a reduction in morbidity or mortality. However, there will also be an associated cost. This cost may be at the expense of the rights or opportunities of a target or a non-target group.

The steps for planning an intervention detailed above are all interlaced with important ethical questions that need to be addressed. The benefits of a public health intervention must be carefully considered. That the intervention itself must be based on sound evidence should not be overlooked as an important ethical consideration. When designing an intervention, programme planners will consider multiple routes of achieving the stated outcomes. If a particular intervention is selected, this will be at the expense of other interventions that could potentially have been chosen. Therefore, resources will be spent on a chosen intervention method at the expense of all the other options that were available. Public health practitioners should be reasonably sure that the intervention they have chosen is supported by evidence and has a reasonable chance of success. Data must substantiate that a given intervention is capable of achieving the aims of the intervention.

Once the method of intervention has been chosen, the potential harms or burdens of the intervention should be identified. Different interventions will have different levels of burden associated with them. Education (see 'capability' above) is a mode of intervention that comes with little burden on the recipient of the message, but simultaneously, it may not be as effective as other types of intervention. Coercion (see 'motivation' above), on the other hand, may be more effective in eliciting change in particular situations; however, this mode of intervention comes with a much greater level of infringement on individual liberties than education on its own (Kass 2001). Therefore, the principles of beneficence and non-maleficence are important considerations when planning public health interventions. This balance of beneficence and non-maleficence is particularly evident when more than one option is available to achieve a given public health outcome. Given the choice between an education approach and a coercion approach, ethically, the intervention planner should choose the option that comes with the fewest harms and burdens to the population, while ensuring that the planned benefits of the intervention can be achieved (Kass 2001). This choice should be supported by the data.

Programmes must be implemented fairly. Targeting specific groups should only be carried out when there is substantial evidence for attaining the benefit of the intervention while ensuring that other groups are not harmed or burdened.

These ethical problems in public health intervention planning are addressed by Kass (2001) by answering the following questions:

What are the public health goals of the proposed program?
How effective is the program in achieving its stated goals?
What are the known or potential burdens of the program?
Can burdens be minimised? Are there alternative approaches?
Is the program implemented fairly?
How can the benefits and burdens of a program be fairly balanced?

Kass (2001)

Further to these ethical principles in public health interventions, there are important additional considerations to make in the context of global health and nutrition. According to Rutstein et al. (2016), societal values and ethical priorities must be reflected in the outcomes, cost-effectiveness and implementation of public health interventions, particularly in resource-poor settings. Societal values vary across the world. The African philosophical tradition of Ubuntu could be translated as 'I am because others are'. In this philosophy, the individual is regarded in the context of a much wider collective human consciousness, underpinned by a fundamental concept of sharing. This sharing is not limited to sharing experiences and physical objects, but extends to spiritual sharing as well. Therefore, when illness occurs in an individual, it is seen as a manifestation of some action within a community. This contrasts with Western concepts of causality in disease; however, the societal values that are carried with the underlying ideology of the community need to be integrated with the diagnosis and treatment of illness for it to be effective. In this African tradition, complete healing cannot be achieved until the patient is able to re-integrate into society. Treatment by healthcare staff is often accompanied by spiritual practices carried out by traditional healers, intended to reconcile the patient with the community and wider collective consciousness (Prinsloo 2001). Rituals or sacrifices may be offered as part of this process. According to Thompson and Wadley (2018), similar principles can be seen in the Pacific, where qualitative evidence suggests that social work is more effective when indigenous practices and traditional values are integrated into practice.

Therefore, using cultural strengths as part of interventions can assist in avoiding two extremes of public health approaches – top-down impositions (such as coercion) and cultural relativism – each of which undermines the potential effectiveness of public health interventions either by reducing the acceptance of a given intervention by a population or by failing to challenge harmful practices (Thompson and Wadley 2018).

The two dominant approaches in public health have been social determinant and rights-based approaches and biomedical or pathogenic approaches (Loewenson et al. 2021). Biomedical approaches were used in sub-Saharan Africa, India and South America under colonial rule, which had the effect of undermining indigenous understandings of health (Loewenson et al. 2021). A shift in health system approach from a medical model that emphasises individual health while considering social organisation of the health system as contributory towards a health economics approach that emphasises the distribution of health in the context of political, social, economic and cultural structures has been taking place (Ichoku et al. 2013). For healthcare systems to succeed in reducing health inequities, they must be modelled around societal values and not simply from inherited mono-cultural paradigms (Ichoku et al. 2013).

10.6 Designing a Logframe Analysis

A logframe analysis is a common requirement when designing and applying for funding for an intervention from international aid agencies. This section presents the concept of the logframe and a worked example.

10.6.1 Designing a Logframe

'Logframe' is shorthand for 'logical framework' and is often required as part of an application for funding public health interventions. The logframe is a tool that focuses on planning, implementing, managing and monitoring a project. The tool requires the public health intervention planner to identify the main elements of an intervention strategy and to make links between these main elements (Department of International Development of the United Kingdom 2002).

A logframe seeks to establish the following questions:

- If activities are implemented, what outputs will be produced?
- If outputs are produced, will outcomes result?
- If outcomes result, will the objectives be achieved?
- Will the outcomes contribute to the larger goal?
- Impact: Set of program results that occur at the **beneficiary level** and can be directly attributed to the program activities rather than external factors.

Impacts and outputs are not the same thing

Impacts	Outputs
Intermediate improvements in capability of beneficiaries to improve their own lives	Refers to quantity and quality of goods and services delivered through program activities
Final improvements in economic and personal well-being of individuals who receive goods and services through the program	

Riely et al. (1999)

Aspects of a logframe are as follows:

- Aim
- Component-specific outcomes
- Objectives
- Strategies
- Outputs
- Outcomes

10.6.2 Example of a logframe

An example of a logframe analysis is given in Figure 10.8. In this instance, an intervention is being proposed which aims to establish antenatal classes (ANC) in an effort to reduce the risk of childhood stunting. In this format, columns are provided for the objectives, strategy, outputs and outcomes.

AIM:
To prevent and address nutritional stunting amongst infants and young children by empowering pregnant women early in gestation through antenatal care (ANC) classes and continued support up to 24 months after delivery

Component-specific outcomes:
- I. Improvement on infant practices
- II. Instilled sense of community and support as well as autonomy and agency through empowerment of young women by increased access to information, skills development and resources
- III. Improved maternal health and pregnancy outcomes for both mother and child

Objectives	Strategies	Output	Outcomes
To improve breast feeding and complementary feeding practices	Establish antenatal classes run by trained 'mentor moms'. Supported by a community health worker(CHW) who provide young pregnant women with a sense of support, as well as information and practical advice on optimal feeding for their infants and young children Improve on the attendance of ANC classes by providing incentives to young women for be present based on a stratified system	Antenatal classes established and maintained, providing support and advice to pregnant women and mothers of infants Improvements made in the number of women successfully breastfeeding exclusively for the first six months of their infants' lives Resulting higher rate of women attending ANC classless earlier into pregnancy	Hold 46 ANC classes monthly 3–20 women attending every ANC class Improvement in the EBF rate as reported as support groups Improved number of women attending ANC before 20 weeks
To improve household food security and increase dietary diversity in a marginalised	Provide trays of eggs to all women attending ANC classes pre-and post-partum weekly or	Increased dietary diversity and inclusion of vegetables and animal protein in	Provide nutritious food (eggs) to 920 people monthly

Figure 10.8: Designing a logframe.

References

Bartholomew, L.K., Parcel, G.S., and Kok, G. (1998). Intervention mapping: a process for developing theory- and evidence-based health education programs. *Health Educ. Behav.* 25: 525–563.

Beauchamp, T.L. and Childress, J.F. (2008). *Principles of Biomedical Ethics*. Oxford: Oxford University Press.

Bell, N. (2008). Ethics in child research: Rights, reason and responsibilities. *Children's Geographies* 6 (1): 7–20.

Brown, T.M., Cueto, M., and Fee, E. (2006). The World Health Organization and the transition from 'international' to 'global' public health. *Am. J. Public Health* 96: 62–72. https://doi.org/10.2105/AJPH.2004.050831.

Campbell, N.C., Murray, E., Darbyshire, J. et al. (2007). Designing and implementing complex interventions to improve health care. *Br. Med. J.* 334: 455–459.

CORE Group (2008). *Designing for Behaviour Change Framework*. Washington: CORE Group and USAID.

De Zoysa, J., Habicht, P., Pelto, G. et al. (1998). Research steps in the development and evaluation of public health interventions. *Bull. World Health Organ.* 76: 127–133.

Department of International Development of the United Kingdom (2002). Tools for Development: A handbook for those involved in development activity.

Green, L. and Kreuter, M.K. (2005). *Health Program Planning: An Educational and Ecological Approach*, 4e. New York: McGraw Hill.

Ichoku, H.E., Mooney, G., and Ataguba, J.E. (2013). Africanizing the social determinants of health: embedded structural inequalities and current health outcomes in sub-Saharan Africa. *Int. J. Health Serv.* 43 (3): 745–759.

Kass, N.E. (2001). An ethics framework for public health. *Am. J. Public Health* 91 (11): 1776–1782.

Lehmann, U. and Sanders, D. (2007). *Community Health Workers: What Do we Know About them? The State of the Evidence on Programmes, Activities, Costs and Impact on Health Outcomes of Using Community Health Workers*. Geneva: World Health Organisation.

Loewenson, R., Villar, E., Baru, R., and Marten, R. (2021). Engaging globally with how to achieve healthy societies: insights from India, Latin America and east and southern Africa. *BMJ Glob. Health* 6 (4): e005257.

Matteson, P.C. (1999). Malaria control in South America. *Emerging Infectious Diseases* 5 (2): 309–310.

MRC (2008). *Development and Evaluation of Complex Interventions: New Guidance*. London: Medical Research Council.

Prinsloo, E.D. (2001). A comparison between medicine from an African (Ubuntu) and Western Philosophy. *Curationis* 24 (1): 58–65.

Riely, F., Mock, N., Cogill, B. et al. (1999). *Food Security Indicators and the Framework for Use in the Monitoring and Evaluation of Food Aid Programs*. Washington: Food and Nutrition Technical Assistance Project (FANTA).

Rutstein, S.E., Price, J.T., Rosenberg, N.E. et al. (2016). Hidden costs: the ethics of cost-effectiveness analyses for health interventions in resource-limited settings. *Glob. Public Health* 12 (10): https://doi.org/10.1080/17441692.2016.1178319.

Thompson, L.J. and Wadley, J. (2018). Integrating indigenous approaches and relationship – based ethics for culturally safe interventions: child protection in the Solomon Islands. *Int. Social Work* 62 (2): 994–1010.

Wight, D., Wimbush, E., Jepson, R., and Doi, L. (2016). Six steps in quality intervention development (6SQuID). *J. Epidemiol. Community Health* 70: 520–525.

World Medical Association (2013). WMA Declaration of Helsinki – Ethical Principles for Medical Research Involving Human Subjects. Available from: https://www.wma.net/policies-post/wma-declaration-of-helsinki-ethical-principles-for-medical-research-involving-human-subjects/

11 Nutrition in Emergencies

The global problem of hunger is most acutely seen in regions facing emergencies, including climate change, armed conflicts and natural disasters. These problems exacerbate the challenges already faced by other regions of the world. Challenges facing the globe include providing enough food to meet the needs of the growing world population and the destruction of natural resources. As the world population continues to grow, the need to produce more food puts additional pressure on the environment and economic and political systems. Solutions to these problems will need to involve food production and distribution, protecting the environment and accounting for the growing global population.

Economic and political issues are drivers of hunger in emergency situations. Fluctuations in food prices and wages and major changes to government policies can result in significant disruptions to food security. This was seen during the Chinese famine during the late 1950s and early 1960s. Radical changes to agricultural policy combined with adverse environmental conditions resulted in approximately 30 million deaths during this period. Economic instability and political volatility in Zimbabwe in the 2000s resulted in hyperinflation. Zimbabwe's gross domestic product contracted by 40% between 2000 and 2008, and inflation increased to greater than 200 million percent. Additionally, 80% of the population was unemployed (Tawodzera 2014). There was a food production deficit of 1 million tonnes for maize, Zimbabwe's staple crop. The country needed approximately 1.8 million tonnes of maize in 2008, of which 1.5 million tonnes were required for human consumption and the remainder for livestock feed (Mudzonga and Chigwada 2009). These factors had a substantial negative effect on household food security.

Armed conflicts are a major cause of famine worldwide. It was estimated that there were 6 million people hungry in Syria in 2015. The nature of the war in this region has made access difficult to impossible for aid workers.

Natural disasters and climate change result in food shortages. The drought in Ethiopia in 2014 placed 15 million people at risk of malnutrition and death. International food relief programmes act as safety nets for countries facing natural disasters.

In regions affected by instability, conflict or natural disasters, food becomes unaffordable, inaccessible and unavailable. This results in inadequate food intake, which does not meet the nutritional and energy requirements for growing children, contributing to undernutrition.

11.1 Climate Change

Simulated climate models developed in the 1980s predicted an approximate increase in global surface temperature of 0.2 °C every 10 years based on greenhouse gas emissions. Subsequent research has demonstrated that the predictions were largely accurate (Hansen et al. 2006). A global temperature increase of greater than 1 °C relative to the year 2000 is considered extremely dangerous, and is likely to result in rising sea levels and mass extinctions.

The El Niño effect is a cyclical rise in ocean temperatures in the equatorial Pacific, which forms part of the larger El Niño Southern Oscillation phenomenon. El Niño events can have dramatic effects on weather conditions across the world, causing flooding in some regions and droughts in others. Warm sea surface temperatures in the equatorial Pacific are associated with dry seasons in Ethiopia and a slower Indian monsoon system (Gleixner et al. 2017). Strong El Niño effects took place in 1983 and 1998. It is thought that increased global temperatures and raised temperatures in the eastern Pacific Ocean in particular will result in more extreme El Niño effects in coming years (Hansen et al. 2006).

Climate change is also predicted to affect water supplies in many regions. A global temperature rise of 1.5 °C is predicted to correspond to a 2 °C rise in the mountainous regions of Asia. This increase in temperature will result in a loss of approximately one-third of the ice mass in these mountains by 2100 (Kraaijenbrink et al. 2017). A 1.5 °C increase in global surface temperatures is considered a conservative prediction, and higher rises in temperature will result in a near depletion of ice in these regions. As the glaciers in the high mountains of Asia are a significant contributor to the water supply of millions of people, the projected loss of glacier ice will have significant consequences for water management for these populations (Kraaijenbrink et al. 2017).

Water security is an important dimension of food security. The impact of climate change, including melting glaciers as well as periods of more severe flooding and droughts in many regions of the world, is expected to affect the quality and quantity of available water for human populations.

As human urban populations grow, challenges in maintaining safe and adequate water supplies increase. The anticipated impacts of climate change are now included in guidelines for planning drinking water supplies. The Stockholm Framework incorporates risk assessment into planning water use and planning regulations and policies on drinking water (WHO 2017).

Food production is being affected by climate change, with implications for the sustainability of the food supply. Higher temperatures have an effect on crop production. Higher night temperatures interfere with plant respiration and produce smaller yields. Divergence from normal seasonal temperatures affects the reproductive cycles of food crops, resulting in diminished yields from otherwise healthy plants (Rasul et al. 2011). Evidence is beginning to emerge that weather events including seasonality, rainfall, temperature are associated with child stunting. This association is mediated by socio-economic, demographic and agricultural factors suggesting that segments of the population are at a higher risk of malnutrition resulting from climate change (Phalkey et al. 2015).

The 'green revolution' that took place following the second World War introduced industrial processes to agriculture on a grand scale, involving monoculturing, widespread reliance on pesticides and fertilisers, and removal of wildlife habitats (Raven and Wagner 2021). This industrialisation of agriculture has been detrimental to species biodiversity and threatening to insect life (Raven and Wagner 2021). Hedgerows have been removed in European agricultural land, while rice fields, which can act as important habitats for wetland species in Asia, were damaged by chemical use from the 1950s to 1970s (Katayama et al. 2015). Pollinators including bees and birds are being lost as agricultural land encroaches on wild lands. In addition to the loss of biodiversity, this is also implicated in the spread of zoonotic diseases, such as COVID-19, as humans and animals are forced to live in closer proximity to each other, increasing the risk of viruses crossing the species barrier.

Wheat, rice, soya beans and maize represent three quarters of the world's available food energy. Commercial crops may not be resistant to local conditions, but a region's native plant species are being lost as they are not commercially viable for foods. Genetic information in local crops may play a role in creating weather-resistant commercial crops. It is widely accepted that climate change will have an impact on staple crop yields. This will affect the amount of food energy available to the human population. However, other crops such as vegetables, legumes and tubers, which are important for dietary diversity, will also be affected by climate change (Scheelbeek et al. 2018). The effects of climate change on food crops will not be limited to the quantity of food produced but are likely to have an impact on their nutritional quality. The amount of protein, iron and zinc found in staple crops is affected by the amount of carbon dioxide in the atmosphere. Projected increases in atmospheric CO_2 over the coming decades could result in an additional 175 million people deficient in zinc, and a decrease in available iron by 4% (Myers and Smith 2018). Countries in South Asia, Africa and the Middle East will experience the greatest impacts of these changes in terms of public health (Myers and Smith 2018).

Changes in global food availability resulting from climate change will affect dietary patterns. It is projected that per capita vegetable and fruit consumption will be reduced by 4% and red meat consumption will be reduced by 0.7% (Springman et al. 2016). Models suggest that these dietary changes will be associated with 529 000 climate-related deaths (Springman et al. 2016).

The food system (Figure 11.1) is a major contributor to climate change and is affected by climate change. Not only will climate change have an effect on the food system, food availability and dietary patterns, but the food system itself contributes to climate change. Limiting the increase in global temperature to the target of 1.5 °C will not be achievable if current trends in global food systems persist, even if fossil fuel emissions halted immediately (Clark et al. 2020). Therefore, meeting the global temperature targets will require changes in non-food industry as well as food industries.

Additional nutrition concerns related to climate change include its impact on migration. There is growing speculation that climate change is already a driver or conflict and migration of human populations.

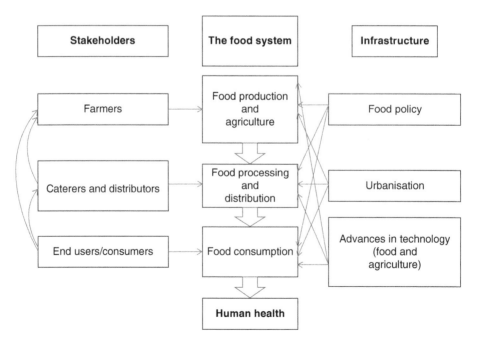

Figure 11.1: The food system revisited.

According to Abel et al. (2019), a causal relationship between climate, conflict and asylum seeking has only recently been established. Consequences of climate change including droughts and resultant crop failure in combination with poor natural resource management cause conflict for resources. This is particularly important when there are already demographic pressures in the area facing conflict. Both conflict and climate change result in an increase in migration away from the affected areas as people leave for better resourced regions. The consequence of this is an increase in internally displaced people and more refugees and asylum seekers leaving their homes (Abel et al. 2019).

11.2 Global Nutrition and Health Strategies in the Context of Climate Change

Environmental enteric dysfunction has been identified as a causative factor in stunting and wasting among children. Enteral pathogens also impact micronutrient status by damaging intestinal villi and through the action of inflammation. The most common water-borne diseases include cholera, typhoid, amebiasis and helminth infestations. These food and water-borne diseases are responsible for many deaths and illnesses across the world. WaSH strategies are often employed to prevent these infections from taking place, as an important nutrition-sensitive intervention in improving nutritional status in endemic areas. It is thought that climate change will impact the effectiveness of these strategies. As flood patterns change as a result of climate change, drinking water sources will be impacted. This could result in a higher burden of water-borne disease. Therefore, strategies such as mapping flood impacts on drinking water sources and robust WaSH strategies will be important aspects of global nutrition and health in the context of climate change (Cisse 2019).

Mapping floods will be an increasingly useful tool in the future. Desertification presents another area where interventions may be effectively targeted. Desertification refers to the degradation of land in arid and semi-arid areas. It is a consequence of human activities and environmental changes. For example, clearing vegetation cover for use for fuel or agriculture removes the protective vegetation that maintains the soil quality and prevents water run-off. This results in the soil degradation known as desertification. According to the United Nations Organisation (2019), 12 million hectares of arable land are lost to desertification every year. Models suggest that the expanding arid zone will contribute to 250 000 cases of stunting and 100 000 cases of anaemia by 2025 (Jankowska et al. 2012). Policymakers have identified desertification as a cause of conflict, fires and unemployment. Identifying areas at risk of this problem and taking steps to prevent it would present a meaningful target for intervention.

Efforts for preventing desertification and reversing its spread include the 'Green Wall' in sub-Saharan Africa and re-forestation in South America. The Green Wall aims to create a green barrier 8000 km long across the width of the African continent and involves more than 20 countries. These efforts have many positive effects, including improved economic activity and women's empowerment in affected communities (United Nations Organisation 2019). Another strategy for improving food security in regions stricken by drought is to develop climate-resilient crops. These climate-resilient crop varieties may help farmers to adapt to the changing climate. Climate-resilient crops may be tolerant to dry conditions or utilise available water more efficiently. However, the uptake of this strategy has been slow (Acevedo et al. 2020). A lack of available outreach and education services hinders the expansion of adopting climate-resilient crops by farmers. Difficulty in accessing seeds and fertilisers are also inhibitors of this approach. Farmers with lower education levels or poorer socio-economic status are less likely to adopt the approach.

Despite a growing trend in the popularity of plant-based diets across the world, the FAO reports that the overall trend in diets is shifting towards consuming animal products including meat, milk and dairy. While beneficial effects have been shown in terms of growth and development from using animal foods high in biologically available proteins, the additional resources required in rearing livestock have a detrimental effect on the environment. All agricultural activities require inputs that drive climate change such as using fossil fuels. However, livestock production is less efficient than plant production and contributes additional greenhouse gas emissions from the animals themselves. Rearing animals for food requires feed so that crops and agricultural land and resources that could be used for human consumption are diverted to producing feeds including crops and fisheries. The benefits of rearing animals, namely economic opportunities, improved food security and dietary diversification, must be balanced against risks to natural resources. The current pace of increase in animal production makes these risks difficult to manage, and land use must be carefully considered (FAO et al. 2018).

11.3 Armed Conflict and Nutritional Emergencies

Armed conflict results in malnutrition among populations. In many cases, food supply lines are disrupted by wars, which leave people vulnerable to food insecurity. Once a nutritional emergency has set in, it is often this poor access that inhibits humanitarian efforts to feed affected populations – medicines and food supplies, including emergency foods used to treat acute malnutrition, are unable to reach people in need. Armed conflict also results in population displacement. For communities that rely on subsistence agriculture for food security, this is especially detrimental. Armed conflicts may also result in sudden economic shocks – currencies may suddenly be worthless than they were before, resulting in greater levels of poverty in a population and difficulties in accessing resources. Normal health services and infrastructure may be interrupted and, in extreme cases, targeted during conflicts.

11.4 Drivers of Humanitarian Emergencies

Signs of approaching humanitarian emergencies are not easy to recognise, but different forms of humanitarian emergency may be the result of particular sources. Stagnation and decline in gross domestic product may precipitate an economic emergency, as may high levels of inflation, income inequality and slow growth in average food production (Auvinen and Nafziger 1999). Violent conflict and large amounts of money spent on the military relative to national income may also be a source of emergencies (Auvinen and Nafziger 1999). Early warning signs of humanitarian crises may be seen by monitoring accelerating factors and decelerating factors associated with crises (Harff and Gurr 1998). It is for this reason that nutrition surveillance is an important aspect of governance.

11.5 Natural Disasters and Nutritional Emergencies

The effects of climate change have been discussed, but these changes are relatively slow in comparison to other natural disasters such as tsunamis, tropical cyclones (hurricanes) and wildfires. The changes brought about by these natural disasters are acute, and effective prevention strategies cannot easily be determined ahead of time through nutritional surveillance. It is important that governments have plans in place for emergency situations and make use of nutritional surveillance systems to anticipate potential consequences and targets should an emergency occur.

Emergencies such as floods resulting from tropical cyclones and tsunamis destroy infrastructure. This includes agricultural infrastructure, which affects food security. It also destroys logistical infrastructure, resulting in difficulties in bringing food in to increase the available supply. In addition, health services are interrupted, and health system infrastructure may be damaged or dysfunctional following a crisis. Floods provide a natural environment for enteric pathogens, which increases the risk of infection with typhoid and dysentery. Malnutrition can result from these conditions, as the integrity of the gut mucosa is affected, resulting in poor absorption of nutrients. Clean, potable water sources may be affected, and the treatment of dehydration becomes challenging. This combination of problems can result in rapid deterioration in vulnerable groups such as infants, children and the elderly.

11.6 Strategies to Address Malnutrition in Emergency Settings

The first priority in emergency settings from a nutritional perspective is to prevent the occurrence of severe acute malnutrition. A high incidence of infectious disease and inadequate dietary intake are commonly seen in emergency situations. These emergency situations may be a result of ecological disaster, armed conflict or economic disaster. Emergency relief approaches need to be designed for the specific situation, as there will be common consequences across different types of emergencies, but no single approach will be effective in all emergency contexts.

11.7 Delivering Nutrition Services During Emergencies

Recommendations on infant feeding during emergencies focus on maintaining and supporting breastfeeding. In the past, aid workers have distributed breastmilk substitute and bottles to mothers and infants to prevent malnutrition; however, current practices attempt to promote and support normal breastfeeding in these situations. UNICEF developed infant breastfeeding strategies for emergency situations following the war in Bosnia in 1994. There is good evidence that breastfed infants have fewer bouts of diarrhoea than formula-fed infants. This may be an important quality in emergency situations. Stress hormones only temporarily affect oxytocin levels – this hormone is needed for the let-down reflex but not for breastmilk production, which is reliant on prolactin. Therefore, even it is possible to breastfeed and maintain milk supply even in emergency situations. Nutrient and energy requirements are higher during lactation. Physiological adaptations increase the amount of nutrients absorbed during lactation; however, breastfeeding mothers will require an additional 500 kcal a day to support their body weight. Therefore, when food rationing is used in emergency situations, pregnant and breastfeeding women should be prioritised, and additional rations supplying an extra 500 kcal a day should be available. UNICEF is involved in providing emergency support for breastfeeding and assisted in 6.5 million cases in emergency settings in 2016. Where infant formula is required, it is involved in helping to ensure ethical distribution of these products.

An essential aspect of emergency nutrition strategies is ensuring that micronutrient deficiencies are prevented and treated. As an example, vitamin A deficiency is known to result in a weakened immune system, therefore putting populations in emergency settings at a higher risk of the disease-malnutrition cycle. Iron deficiency is common across the world and is associated with poor growth and development in children.

In addition to emergency feeding schemes, the United Nations Organisation (2019) has recommended that public policy should aim towards better food security to mitigate the risk of deterioration in population nutritional status in vulnerable communities. Strategies worth implementing include education, school meal programmes, biofortification and mandatory micronutrient fortification strategies.

In addition to these nutrition-specific interventions, WaSH as a nutrition-sensitive intervention needs to be prioritised to prevent diarrhoeal diseases. Providing clean, safe water is an important consideration for emergency responses.

Severe acute malnutrition occurs when these preventative measures fail. Screening for acute malnutrition is essential in emergency settings. It is estimated that 61 000 children younger than five years, and 15 000 women of childbearing age, were screened for acute malnutrition in Sudan in 2016 as the crisis emerged there. Screening procedures follow recommendations, with severe acute malnutrition identified using weight for height and MUAC among children. Severe acute malnutrition is treated using the appropriate pathway for complicated or uncomplicated SAM in emergency settings.

11.8 Conclusion

Humanitarian emergencies occur as a result of natural disaster, armed conflict and economic or political upheaval. The major consequences of these emergencies are social disruption, displacement of people, damage and interruption to infrastructure and normal service provision, as well as food shortages and impacts on the availability of clean, safe water. Preventing acute malnutrition is a priority in emergency nutrition. It is recommended that governments have plans in place to prevent nutritional emergencies from occurring through careful nutritional surveillance. Preventative strategies such as micronutrient fortification and investments in education and agriculture can help to prevent or lessen the severity of emergencies. Protecting micronutrient status is an important part of the emergency nutrition approach, as is protecting and promoting breastfeeding for infants. Providing safe water and implementing WaSH strategies help to prevent morbidity and mortality. Pregnant and lactating women, infants and children must be prioritised in nutritional interventions (Gasseer et al. 2004). Screening for acute malnutrition and treating acute malnutrition appropriately when it is identified must be conducted when preventative measures fail.

11.9 The Future of Nutrition and Global Health

Health workers will be facing new challenges over the course of the twenty-first century. As the population continues to grow and pressure on the environment increases, nutritionists, dieticians, doctors, nurses, farmers, policymakers and others will need to identify new strategies for addressing malnutrition, overnutrition and the environment. Improvements in nutritional screening and surveillance systems will be needed for more accurate and earlier identification of nutritional problems. A deeper understanding of the relationship between the environment and health, including the relationship between diseases, genetics and nutritional status, will be needed to better target interventions. Public health systems will be challenged by rising levels of malnutrition – of undernutrition and micronutrient deficiency – as well as overweight and obesity and the consequences of these conditions in terms of noncommunicable disease burdens. The next decade will see some countries on track to meet the UN Sustainable Development Goals targets, and others falling behind.

References

Abel, G.J., Brottrager, M., Cuaresma, J.C., and Muttarak, R. (2019). Climate, conflict and forced immigration. *Glob. Environ. Chang.* 54: 239–249.

Acevedo, M., Pixley, K., Zinyengere, N. et al. (2020). A scoping review of adoption of climate- resilient crops by small-scale producers in low- and middle-income countries. *Nat. Plants* 6: 1231–1241.

Auvinen, J. and Nafziger, E.W. (1999). The sources of humanitarian emergencies. *J. Confl. Resolut.* 43 (3): 267–290.

Cisse, G. (2019). Food-borne and water-borne diseases under climate change in low- and middle-income countries: further efforts needed for reducing environmental health exposure risks. *Acta Trop.* 194: 181–188.

Clark, M.A., Domingo, N.G.G., Colgan, K. et al. (2020). Global food system emissions could preclude achieving the 1.5° and 2°C climate change targets. *Science* 370 (6517): 705–708.

FAO, IFAD, UNICEF, WFP, WHO (2018). *The State of Food Security and Nutrition in the World 2018. Building climate resilience for food security and nutrition.* Rome: FAO.

Gasseer, N.A., Dresden, E., Keeney, G.B., and Warren, N. (2004). Status of women and infants in complex humanitarian emergencies. *J. Midwifery Womens Health* 49 (S4): 7–13.

Gleixner, S., Keenlyside, N., Viste, E., and Korecha, D. (2017). The El Nino effect on Ethiopian summer rainfall. *Climate Dynam.* 49: 1865–1883.

Hansen, J., Sato, M., Ruedy, R. et al. (2006). Global temperature change. *PNAS* 103 (39): 14288–14293. https://doi.org/10.1073/pnas.0606291103.

Harff, B. and Gurr, T.R. (1998). Systematic early warning of humanitarian emergencies. *J. Peace Res.* 35 (5): 551–580.

Jankowska, M.M., Lopez-Carr, D., Funk, C. et al. (2012). Climate change and human health: spatial modelling of water availability, malnutrition and livelihoods in Mali, Africa. *Appl. Geogr.* 33: 4–15.

Katayama, N., Baba, Y.G., Kusomoto, Y., and Tanaka, K. (2015). A review of post-war changes in rice farming and biodiversity in Japan. *Agr. Syst.* 132: 73–84.

Kraaijenbrink, P.D.A., Bierkens, M.F.P., Lutz, A.F., and Immerzeel, W.W. (2017). Impact of a global temperature rise of 1.5 degrees Celsius on Asia's glaciers. *Nature* 549: 257–260.

Mudzonga, E. and Chigwada, T. (2009). *Agriculture: Future Scenarios for Southern Africa – A Case Study of Zimbabwe's Food Security.* Canada: International Institute for Sustainable Development (IISD).

Myers, S.S. and Smith, M.R. (2018). Impact of anthropogenic CO_2 emissions on global human nutrition. *Nat. Clim. Change* 8: 834–839.

Phalkey, R.K., Aranda-Jan, C., Marx, S. et al. (2015). Systematic review of current efforts to quantify the impacts of climate change on undernutrition. *PNAS* 112 (33): e4522–e4529.

Rasul, G., Chaudhry, Q.Z., Mahmood, A., and Hyder, K.W. (2011). Effect of temperature rise on crop growth and productivity. *Pak. J. Meteorol.* 8 (15): 53–62.

Raven, P.H. and Wagner, D.L. (2021). Agricultural intensification and climate change are rapidly decreasing insect biodiversity. *PNAS* 118 (2): e2002548117. https://doi.org/10.1073/pnas.2002548117.

Scheelbeek, P.F.D., Birda, F.A., Tuomistob, H.L. et al. (2018). Effect of environmental changes on vegetable and legume yields and nutritional quality. *PNAS* 115 (26): 6804–6809.

Springman, M., Mason-D'Croz, D., Robinson, S. et al. (2016). Global and regional health effects of future food production under climate change: a modelling study. *Lancet* 387 (10031): P1937–P1946.

Tawodzera, G. (2014). Household food insecurity and survival in Harare: 2008 and beyond. *Urban Forum* 25: 207–216.

United Nations Organisation (2019). Every year, 12 million hectares of productive land lost, secretary general tells Desertification Forum, calls for scaled- up restoration efforts, small policies. Press release, available from: https://www.un.org/press/en/2019/sgsm19680.doc.htm

WHO (2017). *Guidelines for drinking-water quality, 4th Ed incorporating the first addendum.* Geneva: World Health Organisation.

Index

Nutrition and Global Health, First Edition. Shawn W. McLaren.
© 2023 John Wiley & Sons Ltd. Published 2023 by John Wiley & Sons Ltd.